Thank you for taking this journey with me!

FINISH YOUR RACE

Don Armstrong

FINISH
YOUR RACE

FINISH
YOUR RACE

Empower
Your
Life with
Strategies
from a
**Cancer
Survivor**

DON ARMSTRONG

Published by Empower Life Press

www.DonArmstrongLive.com

ISBN: 978-0-9979166-0-7

Book design by AuthorSupport.com
Cover Photo by Jon Uzzel
Illustrations by Shamsy Roomiani

Printed in the United States of America

First Edition

DEDICATION

*Every three minutes, one person in the United
States is diagnosed with a blood cancer.*

*Every nine minutes, someone in the United
States dies from a blood cancer.*

*Dedicated in memory of the individuals
who lost their battle to blood cancer.*

*Dedicated in honor of the survivors who are living
with, or who are in remission from, blood cancer.*

*Dedicated to the individuals—doctors, researchers, the
Leukemia & Lymphoma Society's staff, and volunteers—
who are committed to finding a cure for blood cancer.*

MY COMMITMENT

The Leukemia & Lymphoma Society's mission: cure leukemia, lymphoma, Hodgkin's disease, and myeloma and improve the quality of life of patients and their families.

Since being diagnosed with leukemia in 2005, I've learned of the groundbreaking work done by LLS. I am confident that the work done by LLS is in part responsible for me being alive today. As a result, I am dedicated to raising awareness and research dollars for LLS. Toward that objective, a portion of the proceeds from **Finish YOUR Race** *will be donated to the Leukemia & Lymphoma Society to support the organization's mission.*

Table of Contents

Acknowledgments

This book has been five years in the making. There were times when I doubted it would be completed. However, there was always someone or something that kept me going. I didn't write this book alone. There were a number of people who helped me along the way. I would like to recognize and acknowledge those who got me to the finish line.

Claudia Read (Getting Organized), you've been with me since day one. You embraced my message and helped me put pen to paper. You never gave up on me or the notion that I had a message to share. I remember you saying, "The world is waiting for you to finish this book." Thank you!

Ann McIndoo and the team at *7 Easy Steps to Write Your Book*, thank you for giving me the tools to get words from my head to paper. Your system, from the Author's Manuscript Grid, Trigger Sentences, Chapter Development, and more, was invaluable in getting content for my book in black and white. I am grateful for your assistance.

Jessica Llanes, you showed me how to take my ideas and turn them into sentences that became paragraphs, eventually chapters, and ultimately a book. Thank you for your calming words and gentle encouragement. Your advice was always helpful! Thank you, my friend.

A big thank you to Steve Harrison and his amazing team at Bradley Communications Corp. and the Quantum Leap program, in particular Martha Bullen, Deb Englander, and Geoffrey Berwind, for keeping me on track. I had no idea there were so many nuances to writing and finishing a book. The support provided by your team helped me understand and put the pieces together. Thank you for smoothing the way for me.

Lindsey Alexander (The Reading List), your experience, expertise, support, and guidance made this book come alive. I appreciate your diligence in helping me get my thoughts and words into what I now proudly call *Finish YOUR Race*. Thank you! Thank you! Thank you!

Lisa Kruczynski (Kruczynski Consulting), you were always in the mix working on developing my website, taking care of all things involving social media, marketing, promotion, and so much more. Your guidance and support on so many levels is appreciated. Knowing you are part of the team is important to me. Thank you for helping make my plans a reality.

Special thank you to Sandie Rodda, Dianna Bryan, Patricia Thomson, and Steve Armstrong for taking time out of your busy lives to read through my manuscript. I appreciate your dedication to scrutinizing every word and sentence. Your feedback and suggestions were important to the final product.

Jon Uzzel, thanks for the genius you expressed in taking my cover photo. You made me a believer. Your eye and sense of what works is appreciated.

Jerry Dorris (AuthorSupport.com), your expertise in pulling all the parts of this book together in preparation for publishing are appreciated. Thank you for the attention to detail.

Julie Bermudez, your willingness to offer your talents in the area of graphic design is appreciated. Every detail counts, and your assistance was an important part of the final product. Thank you!

Shamsy Roomiani, I wanted the pages of this book to be interesting and inviting to the reader. Your illustrations at the beginning of each chapter delivered and met my expectations. Thank you!

Dave Yeager, I appreciate your extraordinary proofreading and copyediting skills. Thank you for your timeliness in bringing clarity to the final manuscript and giving me the confidence to say, "I am done!"

Terri Holiday, thank you for always encouraging me and, yes, pushing me to "get your book done!" You have no idea how much I appreciate your support and love! Thanks to you, I am holding *Finish YOUR Race* in my hands!

One more acknowledgment to Claudia Read. Thank you for hanging with me for five years. Thank you for your prayerful guidance and sharing in my desire to write an impactful book. I appreciate you believing in me and this project. We succeeded, and for that I am grateful for your support. Thank you, my friend.

Finally, I thank God every day for the chance to be a survivor and a thriver of life.

This book would not have been possible without the individuals above. To say this was a team effort is an understatement. This book is a testament to dedication, diligence, and a never-give-up attitude. It's all about *Finish YOUR Race*!

Introduction

On a blustery Texas morning in December 2010, as a cold wind whipped across the course, reddening my already wind-chapped face, I labored into the last mile of the White Rock Marathon in Dallas. Though my feet hurt and my knees ached, I picked up the pace as the finish line came into view. This was the third marathon in three weekends and the end of my yearlong Finish Your Race campaign that had taken me all around the United States. During that long final mile, I reflected on the cities I'd visited, the amazing individuals I'd met, the support and encouragement I'd received, and the challenges I'd overcome. I felt an exhilarating rush of joy for what I had accomplished, along with a bit of sadness that this journey was coming to a close. I laughed, I cried, I winced in pain, and yet I still had a spring in my step as I crossed the finish line, cold and tired but deeply satisfied. I'd finished this race with a newfound confidence and was looking forward to continuing the race of my life.

Five years earlier, as I sat in my room at Baylor's Sammons Cancer Center waiting for the second round of chemo to start, at the beginning of another thirty-day hospital stay, I would have been grateful to run just half a mile—forget about 26.2 miles. I'd been diagnosed with acute myeloid leukemia (AML), a blood cancer. Statistically speaking, my outlook wasn't great. In fact, early in my cancer journey I learned that fewer than 30 percent of those diagnosed with AML survive beyond five years. Following my first round of chemo, my oncologist explained that a stem cell transplant could improve my prognosis; however, a donor needed to be found. In the meantime, more chemo was necessary to keep my cancer in remission. The longest ten months of my life were those I endured fighting for my life, uncertain of what my future would hold, while waiting for a donor.

It has now been over ten years since I was diagnosed with leukemia. During this time, I have been blessed with incredible experiences and moments of true understanding about the world around me. I have raised thousands of dollars for the Leukemia & Lymphoma Society (LLS) and become an outspoken advocate for the organization. I'm now a marathon coach for Team in Training (TNT), I cofounded a nonprofit race (Honored Hero Run) raising over $135,000 for blood cancer research, and as a public speaker and author I'm committed to sharing my experiences. My health—physically and emotionally—has been transformed since that frightening conversation with my doctor a decade ago, however, finding my way to where I am now was by no means easy.

In 2010, I celebrated my fifth year of survivorship from leukemia. This was a milestone year for me, and I wanted to do something extraordinary to mark the occasion. I decided to run five half marathons and five full marathons with Team in Training, the Leukemia

& Lymphoma Society's endurance training program, to raise awareness about blood cancer and money to fund research for a cure. This campaign was intended as a yearlong journey; in the span of twelve short months, however, it became much more.

I chose the title "Finish Your Race" for my 2010 campaign for a simple reason: Life is a journey, and we all have our own course to run, despite the crossroads and crosswinds we encounter along the route. As a survivor, it is my hope that through this book others will find their race and succeed in their own way.

Battling cancer was a true eye-opener for me. It taught me a great deal about myself and about life in general. Prior to my diagnosis, just like many of you, I'd been wrapped up with the activities of simply trying to get by from one day to the next. I thought that was "living," when I had no idea what living really meant. Though I never would have anticipated the outcome as I sat in my hospital room at Baylor, cancer changed almost everything about me for the better. My unexpected transformation began as the impact of leukemia on my life opened my eyes to who I am as a person and what motivates me. What I discovered changed the direction of my life, my priorities, and what I consider today to be important and relevant.

Though I made it through my fight with leukemia, I don't know that the journey ever ends. Surviving has given me a second chance to choose how I live each and every day. Not just surviving but *thriving*! For me, thriving is about being empowered to make changes in spite of everything holding me back—emotionally, physically, mentally, and spiritually—to become my own success story. I try to live every day to the fullest with few, if any, regrets. Most importantly for me, I strive every single day to make a difference in other people's lives. That's my mission, plain and simple.

I don't consider myself a remarkable or exceptional person. Like most of you, I've experienced both good times and not-so-good times. That's part of life! I'd never thought about life as a race until I was diagnosed with a life-threatening disease. Like you, my life's race has led me to a number of pivotal moments that have changed the course and direction of my future. Maybe you're at one of those major crossroads right now, and you don't know how you got there or what to do next. Setbacks in my life and yours can appear in the form of illness, job loss, bankruptcy, divorce, the death of a loved one, and more. For me, it was cancer. Perhaps you've received frightening news about your health recently, or you want to support someone who has had a similar scare. You might be going through a challenging time with a friend or family member, or trying to navigate new and uncertain territory in a relationship. It might be as simple—or as complicated—as this: Today you're not at all where you thought you would be five, ten, twenty years ago.

This book has been five years in the making. I wouldn't want anyone to go through what I did with cancer, yet I do want to share what I learned along the way. If nothing else, I realized this: It is *never* too late to make a difference in yourself and others. With courage, focus, and a positive spirit, you *can* finish your race.

CHAPTER 1

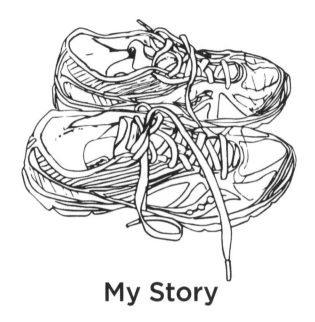

My Story

"Everyone is necessarily the hero of his own life story."

—John Barth

When I was twelve, in 1968, my dad, a fighter pilot in the Air Force, learned he was going to be deployed to Vietnam. It was a scary time for my family, for obvious reasons. Before he left, I remember Dad sitting me down and saying, "Donnie, you're the man of the house while I'm gone." As I understood it, it would be up to me to help keep things together for my mom, older sister, and younger brother. And, in my twelve-year-old mind, I thought, how better to do that than to get a job? After all, that's what the "man of the house" was supposed to do, right?

This may sound farfetched, but I really wanted to work, and I wanted, more than anything, a job at the golf course in our Las Vegas neighborhood. Dad had introduced me to the game of golf when I was ten, and I was immediately hooked. I started to hang around Winterwood Golf Course almost every day, so I had the chance to meet and talk with the managers. One day, I finally summoned the courage to ask golf professional Dick Huff for a job.

Probably because I was so young, Mr. Huff hesitated. He had an opening on his staff, however, he didn't think I was big enough to do all the work the job required. At one point, I remember him telling me, "You can't even see over the golf shop counter. How do you expect to work here?" I was disappointed, to say the least, but I wasn't going to give up. Even after Mr. Huff told me "No", I kept asking for the job. Years later, I realized I was probably something of a pest around Winterwood, but at the time, I didn't think I had anything to lose.

After spending most of a hot summer day at the course, I returned home to find my mom waiting for me at the door. "Mr. Huff called and wants to see you," she told me. As I anxiously walked back to the golf course, I wondered if I had done something wrong. Mr. Huff brought me into his small, cramped office and asked me to sit down. He said that I probably wasn't big enough to handle the position he had available, yet for some reason he couldn't explain to me, he wanted to give me a try. Even though I heard him say, "You've got the job," I insisted on showing him that I could do the job by giving him an eager demonstration of my cart washing and cleaning skills. Recalling that day, he chuckled at how enthusiastic I was to show him I'd work hard. "I never had to tell you something more than once," he told me.

I quickly discovered that I got tremendous satisfaction out of working. At the same time, I was developing a love for the game of golf. In fact, I couldn't get enough of golf, and I practiced before school, after school, and on weekends. At one point, I bought an artificial hitting mat so I could practice chipping in the upstairs hallway of our house late into the evening. I'm sure this drove my parents crazy, but they never said a word about it. When I wasn't playing golf or practicing at home, I was working at the course. Remembering this time, my mom told me, "I never had to think twice about where you were."

> I learned to work hard, apply myself, take direction, and always ask for more responsibility, which for me equaled success.

My first job taught me about work ethic. I learned to work hard, apply myself, take direction, and always ask for more responsibility, which for me equaled success. I was also learning that I could achieve what I set out to accomplish and persistence pays off.

Thankfully, my dad returned from Vietnam, and as planned, we lived in Las Vegas for another three years before he learned he was being transferred to the Pentagon. Before we headed to the East

Coast, I asked Mr. Huff what it would take to have a future in the golf business. He took out a sticky note and wrote two words on it: "Agronomy/Business." I had no idea what agronomy was and didn't know much about business. Mr. Huff explained that agronomy is the science of growing grass on a golf course. He assured me that if I studied both subjects in college, I would be in demand in the golf business when I graduated.

In 1977, I got my degree in agronomy from Virginia Tech, where I minored in business. Not long after, I was offered, and accepted a job at Colonial Country Club in Fort Worth, Texas, as an assistant golf course superintendent. Steve Barley, my second mentor in life, saw something in me and decided to give me a chance. I almost couldn't believe it. Colonial was among the top 100 golf courses in the United States. I watched the Colonial National Invitational golf tournament on TV every year and remembered Ben Hogan had won the tournament five times. I worked hard, applied myself, took direction, and asked for more every single day for the next three years.

Following my early work experience at Colonial, I was offered and accepted golf course superintendent jobs at two different golf courses in the Dallas/Fort Worth area. Twelve months after leaving Colonial, in May 1982, I was asked back as the golf course superintendent. This was a dream job, and at twenty-six years old I was at one of the top country clubs in my profession. I was on cloud nine and determined to take advantage of this opportunity. I worked hard, applied myself, took direction (not much), and asked for more every single day for the next six years.

I was thrilled to be associated with Colonial. In the golf world everyone knew the name, so for me it was exciting to show up to work every day. I loved my work and really enjoyed seeing (almost instantly) the results of my efforts. Of course, I was aware that growing grass in the Texas summer heat can be demanding; however, I was up to the challenge. For me, the bonus was the annual PGA Tour event. I took pride in preparing the golf course to be in top condition for PGA Tour professionals and the golf world to enjoy.

To say I was dedicated to my work was an understatement. I operated with one single goal in mind: to be the best at my profession. I worked hard, and I pressed those who worked with me harder. I got the job done, but I also got used to working seven days a week. My work became something of an obsession. It never even dawned on me that I had lost sight of just about everything else in my life. I was succeeding at my job while making a nice living. In my mind that had to count for something and surely made everything else okay. At least that was my justification. However, I was failing in my personal life, with one unsuccessful marriage and one on less than good terms.

After six years at Colonial, it was time to look for another challenge. I decided to leave one of the most prestigious golf course superintendent jobs in the country and start a golf course consulting company, Golf Resources, Inc. I was fortunate to have outstanding partners, including PGA Tour professional D.A. Weibring, my mentor Steve Barley, new business associate Sam Swanson, and golf legend Byron Nelson. Adhering to my strategy of working hard, taking direction, and asking for more responsibilities, for the next thirteen years, I traveled the world (upward of 150,000 miles per year) consulting on golf projects. Work was all consuming, and yet it was great fun.

But while I was succeeding in my profession and making plenty of money, my life at home was a mess. By this time, my third wife and I weren't seeing eye-to-eye. Sadly, I felt myself growing distant from her daughter and my son. Even though I was traveling the world doing something I truly enjoyed, I was feeling pressure from my wife to be more present in our marriage. If I was going to make my marriage work, I knew I'd need to spend more time at home closer to my family.

This was a significant choice for me as it would mean leaving the industry I had known my entire life, but I chose my family instead of work. I decided to step away from the golf business in June 2000 and jump headfirst into a new endeavor in the financial services industry. In my mind, it wasn't much of a leap, as I believed my previous professional experiences had provided me with a skill set that was well-suited for my newfound industry. Plus, I'd been interested in this industry for years and had studied it in great detail. I believed and justified that I would enjoy the business and was convinced that I could make more money on a schedule that didn't require much traveling. I interviewed with a number of firms in Fort Worth and decided on one I hoped would fit my needs and provide direction. This firm offered training along with the opportunity to be licensed as a financial services representative. Again, I worked incredibly hard and kept asking for more work every single day for the next four years. My efforts started to pay off, but I didn't like the daily scrutiny from management.

In June 2004, I launched my own financial services company. I was done with the corporate side of an industry I wasn't sure suited me long term. I wanted to be on my own without someone telling me when and where I needed to be on a daily basis. But soon, I was working like a crazy person and just not having much success. I was struggling financially in an industry I was actually beginning to dislike, and my home life wasn't improving either. However, quitting is not in my DNA, and I decided to stick with it. Years earlier, I'd learned from Mr. Huff that there are two types of people in the world: Thinkers and Doers. Thinkers contemplate doing something while Doers make things happen. I was determined to be a Doer.

By the following year, in addition to my day job, I had taken on two part-time jobs to pay my bills. I worked almost every waking hour of the day and night. After my regular job, from five p.m. until eight p.m., Monday

> I'd learned from Mr. Huff that there are two types of people in the world: Thinkers and Doers.

through Friday, I sold newspaper subscriptions for the *Fort Worth Star-Telegram*. Then from one a.m. to five a.m., I worked as a newspaper carrier. Seven days a week! By eight a.m. (weekdays), I'd be wearing my financial services hat again. Throwing newspapers was easy, and the route paid decent money, but I was exhausted. Most nights, I was lucky to get more than three hours of sleep.

As a husband, I assumed that my role in my marriage was to solve problems and provide for my family's needs, so I focused on work almost exclusively. In true "man of the house" fashion, I was convinced I was doing everything possible to make ends meet, and if I could make ends meet, everything else would come together. So why wasn't it working? I hadn't even considered the impact my extreme work ethic had on my wife and kids. I just did what I had to, and that had to be enough. Yet in my heart, I knew something had to change. It's just that I had no idea where to start. At forty-nine years old, I was in a moment of crisis and knew nothing of the road ahead.

IN THE BLINK OF AN EYE

There's a song by the Christian rock band MercyMe, "In the Blink of an Eye," that resonates with me. The song refers to the short time we all have on Earth and the fact that things can change quickly and dramatically without warning.

I was too busy trying to succeed in life to notice the warning signs of anything wrong in my body. I had no inkling that I might be ill. It didn't help that my male wiring, combined with an acute type-A personality, further complicated my logic regarding an illness. I truly believed that cancer—or anything else as devastating, for that matter—would never happen to me. Then, the unthinkable happened!

> I was too busy trying to succeed in life to notice the warning signs of anything wrong in my body.

Through the grace of God, on Friday, September 9, 2005, I was visiting with two of my financial services clients, administrators at the James L.

West Alzheimer's Center in Fort Worth. It was the end of a long week of enrolling James L. West employees in a retirement plan. That afternoon, Susan Ferris, the executive director, motioned me into her office first and asked if I was feeling okay.

"You look like a patient with heart problems," she said. I was a bit shocked and asked her to explain. "You look very pale. Do you have anything else going on?"

I did, actually. I rolled up my pant leg to show her what I thought was a rash. She explained that the rash was actually something called petechia, basically a localized hemorrhage that appears as a minute reddish or purplish spot in skin. She was adamant that I get it checked out.

A short time later, as I was leaving for the day, Kay Sharp, the director of nursing, grabbed me in the hallway and ushered me into her office.

"Are you okay?" she asked. "You look horrible."

It was just too strange to ignore: Two women, on the very same day, independently of each other, raised a red flag about my health. Because of their concern, these two amazing, caring women, my guardian angels, started the process that ultimately saved my life.

In the blink of an eye, the journey I thought I was on—working hard, earning a living, and succeeding professionally—took a major detour. I guess I should've known something was wrong. There were symptoms that something wasn't quite right: shortness of breath, light-headedness, fatigue. But frankly, I was just too busy to stop and deal with them. I thought of myself as healthy, despite the breakneck pace of my days. I was active and always on the go. Didn't that mean I was okay? I had bigger, more pressing priorities than pausing to check in with my body, and I believed cancer was something that happened to other people.

It would never happen to me, right?

THE DIAGNOSIS

Though I didn't know it then, those two short conversations late on a Friday afternoon would change my life forever. I knew these women had considerable experience observing people with health issues, and more importantly, I realized they were concerned for me. I remember sitting in my car, calling my wife to tell her about these two unnerving conversations. She didn't hesitate with a response: "For once in your life Don, listen to these conversations and do something about the situation." In a move that was totally out of character for me, I called my primary care physician late that afternoon, after business hours, to set up an appointment for the following Monday.

I was still fairly confident that nothing was wrong with me as I headed to my Monday morning appointment. Surely Dr. Johnson, my primary care doctor for over fifteen years, would confirm this thinking. He asked me several questions about how I was feeling and drew some blood. "*Just a routine visit*," I thought. Then, as I was leaving, Dr. Johnson uncharacteristically followed me to the waiting room and told me, as I walked out the door, "I am concerned about you." Although it struck me as a strange comment in the moment, I was busy and had to get going.

Early the next morning, I was surprised to receive a call from Dr. Johnson himself, instead of one of the nurses. He didn't waste any time: "I got your test results back from the lab, and the results are not good. I think you may have leukemia." "*No way!*" I thought. Time, as it turned out, was of the essence, so much so that he had already made an appointment for me with an oncologist—whom I'd see within the hour. In fact, Dr. Johnson told me he would take me himself if I even thought about hesitating. There was no time for me to think about going. "You've got to go now!" He urged.

My appointment with the oncologist was short—only four or five minutes. Without delay, he sent me to the emergency triage area at Harris Southwest Hospital. For the next twelve hours, I was subjected to a battery of tests to determine my diagnosis. It was here that I had my first experience with a bone marrow aspiration and biopsy. These two tests are done at the same time and, I would later understand, determine whether blood cancer is present.

> I got your test results back from the lab, and the results are not good. I think you may have leukemia.

The triage nurses were terrific and tried to keep things positive. Everything was so new and out of the ordinary for me that I didn't realize at first what they were doing or why. I had two or three nurses working on me at one time, trying to get an intravenous line in one of my veins. They tried for several hours, alternating back and forth, but just couldn't find a vein to access. I thought to myself, "*Why are they working so hard to get a line in?*" I learned later that my body was so anemic (deficient in red blood cells) that finding a usable vein was next to impossible.

At around ten o'clock that night, an overly confident young doctor came charging in to see me. I had no idea why he was there, but he was obviously on a mission. There was one nurse standing at the foot of my bed who'd been in the room with me most of the time.

"He's not ready," she told the doctor. "We've not been able to get a line in him."

The doctor came over to me, patted me on the arm, and said, "He's a tough guy. No problem. We'll just do this."

At that exact moment, I didn't understand what "this" meant, but I sensed the nurse was panicking. Only later did I realize the nurses were trying to put a line in me in an effort to sedate me. Now they were clearly distressed because I was about to undergo a painful procedure without any anesthesia. The doctor asked me to lie down on the bed on my stomach. He used lidocaine to numb the skin around my hip bone. He proceeded to push a hollow needle through the thin skin covering my hip.

As the needle made its way through muscle into my hip bone and eventually into the bone marrow, the pain was indescribably excruciating. At one point, I tried to reach back and grab the doctor by his neck tie to get him to stop. I was unsuccessful in this attempt, and he didn't stop until he had a sample of the liquid portion of the bone marrow (aspiration). As a part of the procedure, he removed a small piece of the bone marrow tissue (biopsy) to complete the process. As the doctor was wrapping up his work, I glanced at the nurse, who was practically in tears.

A few minutes later, my wife passed the doctor in the hallway as he was leaving my room. She asked the doctor, "How did my husband do?" "He did well," the doctor told her. "That's great!" she said, "Because I heard someone in the triage area screaming!" It wasn't long until she discovered that I was the one who'd been screaming. This would be the first of many bone marrow aspirations and biopsies I would receive, but thankfully, the rest weren't nearly as painful.

The following morning, Wednesday, September 14, I was back in the oncologist's office. My official diagnosis was in: acute myeloid leukemia (AML – cancer of the bone marrow and blood). Slowly, the diagnosis started to sink in. I remember thinking, *I have cancer!* but not really being able to process it. This

> I was trying to formulate a plan but didn't really know what to think or do.

was not what I thought I would hear. I sat in my car with my wife in front of the oncologist's office in total silence. Like always, I was trying to formulate a plan but didn't really know what to think or do. Instinctively, I reached for my phone. Without hesitating, my wife asked, "You're calling Rita, aren't you?" I nodded and dialed the number of my good friend who had gone through treatment for AML three years earlier.

I hoped this call would expand my very limited understanding of leukemia, and it did. Once we hung up, I rushed home from the oncologist's office and went directly to my computer. When I landed on a page that defined AML, a single phrase jumped off the screen at me, as if in flashing neon: "Survival rate: 30%." In shock, I turned off the computer, sat back in my chair, and decided I didn't need to read any more. After all, I was about to learn far more about leukemia than I ever imagined.

CHAPTER 2

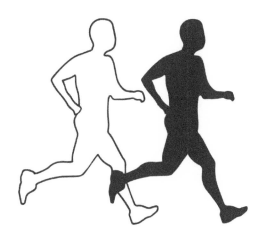

My Race Against Leukemia

*"We shall draw from the heart of suffering itself
the means of inspiration and survival."*

—Winston Churchill

Following my diagnosis, things started to move very quickly. My oncologist wanted me to check in at Harris Hospital immediately. He told me there was a room waiting for me. I chose instead to go home. I needed time, even if it was just twenty-four hours, to bring my family and friends up to date, and to consider my next move. My friend Rita Eatherly had been treated at MD Anderson in Houston, and when I called her she'd been adamant that this hospital was my best option. I was unsure and called Dr. Johnson for his opinion. He agreed that MD Anderson was an excellent choice, but his next words brought my situation into clear focus: "Don, it can take up to two weeks to be admitted to MD Anderson. Let me be perfectly clear: You don't *have* two weeks." For the first time, I understood the seriousness of my illness.

The next morning, Thursday, September 15, I checked into Harris Hospital in downtown Fort Worth at eight a.m. My first day in the hospital went by in a blur. There were so many things happening around me. I'd never really enjoyed being in a hospital. Okay, let's be real, I *hated* being in the hospital. I can't pin this feeling down exactly, I just didn't like it. Of course, whenever I had been in the hospital before, it had been to visit someone, but even those rare experiences made me uncomfortable.

> Let me be perfectly clear: You don't have two weeks." For the first time, I understood the seriousness of my illness.

From the moment I stepped out of the elevator on the seventh floor, it seemed that everyone was moving at hyperspeed. From my vantage point, it appeared the nurses were buzzing up and down the halls, popping in and out of patient rooms. There was constant chatter over the PA system, calls for doctors and nurses to report to specific rooms STAT (immediately). And for me, the smell of rubbing alcohol was so strong I could almost taste it.

Out of the chaos of my first few minutes on the floor, I was introduced to Tracye McNulty, my first oncology nurse. She walked my wife and me to room 729, my home away from home for a while. She talked about the seventh floor and what I could expect over the next several weeks. Tracye had been an oncology nurse for ten years and possessed a wealth of knowledge and experience about leukemia. She was very upbeat and comforting, considering the circumstance and the journey ahead for me. We chatted for a good thirty minutes before she said, "Oh, I guess we should put one of those hospital bracelets on you. Wouldn't want you to get lost." I laughed! I couldn't have asked for a better ambassador, and she brought much-needed relief to a situation that was mind numbing in so many ways.

Following this brief respite, I was jolted back to the reality of the moment as a nurse came into the room to check my blood pressure and vital signs, again. After that, there was one procedure after another: more blood tests, more biopsies, medications to prepare me for chemo—it went on and on.

The nurses seemed to be in a hurry to start treatment, or at least that's how it felt to me. I sensed the seriousness of my illness by the deliberate actions of the nurses. They were trying to be sensitive to my feelings and get me settled in, but they also wanted to get the chemo started as soon as possible. There were more questions to answer, tests to take, and papers to sign. By noon, I had a PICC (peripherally inserted central catheter) line in

> In less than a week, I'd gone from a healthy (or so I'd thought) man to a patient with a life-threatening disease.

my left arm and chemo running through my veins. All the activity made my head spin. In less than a week, I'd gone from a healthy (or so I'd thought) man to a patient with a life-threatening disease.

Still, from that very first day, even as I was adjusting to the idea that I had cancer, I was determined to fight and beat AML. My instinct was to do everything possible—physically, emotionally, mentally, and spiritually—to overcome this disease. The fight part of my fight-or-flight response kicked in—hard.

It helped that, from day one, I had an overwhelming amount of support from family and friends. This support and my faith helped to take the edge off the craziness of the days that followed. My wife was an important part of this support. She was with me every single second and refused to leave my side. In fact, she slept in my room on a chair bed every night of my stay at Harris. She showed remarkable courage throughout this difficult time. She remained upbeat and encouraging, and never showed a moment of doubt. This show of strength was uplifting to me. I can't adequately express how much her love and care meant to me.

The morning of my second day in the hospital, I awoke with a sense of calm as the chaos of the previous day dissipated. I heard in my spirit a voice that clearly told me, "Everything is going to be okay. It will not always be easy, but you will be okay. I have more things for you to do." In those early hours, I truly believe God spoke to me. In that moment, I was infused with an immediate sense of calm, as if a burden had been lifted from my mind. This feeling prevailed with me throughout my treatment. I had a tremendous team of doctors, encouragement from family and friends, and God to guide me through this challenge. I was in a good place as my second day of treatment started.

It's difficult to describe the month I spent in the hospital. So much happened. Some days went by quickly, while some days seemed to never end. I was confined to the seventh floor for my entire stay, which was difficult for someone who was used to coming and going at will in my regular day-to-day life. This floor was occupied primarily by blood cancer patients, a significant number of whom were leukemia patients. Tracye explained that leukemia patients are usually in the hospital for three to four weeks. The seventh floor provided a safe, infection-free environment. Occasionally, I would see an overflow patient from the surgical floor who would stay for two or three days. This was the exception and not the rule.

Chemo shuts off the body's normal ability to produce blood products. My doctor compared the process to a factory shutting down. As a result, secondary infections are a major concern due to a patient's compromised immune system. In fact, more patients die from a secondary infection than from the onset cancer. This is part of the reason patients undergoing 24/7 chemo, like I was, must stay in the hospital long enough for the body to recover from the chemo and resume the process of making blood again.

> Chemo shuts off the body's normal ability to produce blood products. My doctor compared the process to a factory shutting down.

At Harris, I had a private room with a bathroom, and out the window I could see downtown Fort Worth. I spent a significant amount of time staring out that window. Or at the very least, sitting in the chair by the window, feeling the warmth of the sun while I read. There wasn't much fraternizing among the patients, as they were in all stages of treatment. Some patients were doing well, while others were not. Not a terrific social setting. We weren't really prepared or in a position to talk about our own situation to each other.

The nurses were fantastic and a nonstop source of joy, fun, conversation, and counseling. I would spend twelve hours per day (they worked twelve-hour shifts) with a nurse so we became friends. We laughed and cried together many times throughout my stay. I had a constant stream of visitors including family and friends. Friends came from work, church, life—so many of them that I got a guest book to record all their names. It was odd (and certainly unexpected) that some people I thought would surely come to visit me didn't, and then people who I never imagined would stop by to see me regularly. As my journey continued, I appreciated both of those reactions by others to my hospital stay. I understood how difficult it must have been for those who couldn't make it to visit me. I was more than grateful for every single person who took the time to come by. It made the days more normal.

My first round of chemo was successful, and I was released from the hospital in full remission following my thirty-plus-day stay. I was so naïve, I had to ask, "Is being in remission good?" As I hoped, the answer was, "Yes".

When I stepped through the hospital doors, I felt as though I was being released from captivity. In a way, I was. The intense feeling of freedom was something I had never experienced before. I took in all the sights, sounds, and smells of the town I knew so well, as if I was experiencing it for the very first time. There was a strangeness to the drive home, like I'd never traveled those streets before. I was reconnecting with my world again. When I got home, I found my favorite chair, sat down, and sighed.

"So, what's next?" I thought to myself.

THE DONOR SEARCH

After recovering at home for several weeks, I returned to the Harris Hospital for round two of chemo. The nurses greeted me with hugs and were quick to tell me I would be in the same room I'd been in during my first round of chemo. In a peculiar way, this was oddly comforting. I was anxious to get started (and be finished) with round two, but before I could settle in, a call came from Dr. Redrow, my oncologist, to stop the check-in process. He wanted to talk with me about the next steps.

I wasn't sure I understood the previous steps, much less the next steps, but I was all ears. Dr. Redrow explained that I would be a good candidate for a stem cell transplant to eliminate the possibility of leukemia recurring in my future. This was the first time I'd heard the term "stem cell transplant." Essentially, stem cells are basic human cells that reproduce or replicate easily, providing a continuous source of new, sometimes different, types of cells. In a transplant, stem cells are taken from a cancer-free person to replace unhealthy cells in a patient with cancer. A stem cell transplant allows a patient to receive a much higher dose of chemo to kill cancer cells.

Dr. Redrow recommended that I transfer to Baylor Sammons Cancer Research Center, one of the top stem cell transplant centers in the United States. There, the search for a donor began almost immediately. Baylor accessed the *Be the Match Registry* (BTM) to determine the list of potential donors. BTM's registry is the world's largest and most diverse registry of potential marrow donors, now with more than 10.5 million potential donors. BTM partners with international and cooperative registries to provide access to more than 20.5 million potential donors worldwide. Transplant matches are made when a patient's human leukocyte antigen (HLA) and a donor's HLA closely match. I hoped that my sister or brother would be a match, as this would minimize any possible transplant consequences. I was told there was only a 25% chance either of them would be a match, so when they weren't, I wasn't surprised or disappointed. The preliminary donor search showed a list of around a hundred potential donors. That seemed like a good number to me, but I wasn't really sure.

After a few days at Baylor, Dr. Fay, my new oncologist, sat down with me to describe in great detail the pros and cons of a stem cell transplant. On the pro side, the transplanted stem cells engraft into the body and produce the blood products your body requires. The cons, however, are numerous and include side effects from the intense pre-transplant chemo, severe and possibly fatal infection due to a compromised immune system as the body adjusts to the new stem cells, and graft-versus-host disease (GVHD), which occurs when the immune cells from the donor perceive the recipient's body as foreign. GVHD reactions can range from barely noticeable to life threatening.

In the course of the conversation, I was faced with a moment of truth and decision. As Dr. Fay explained it, for some patients a stem cell transplant is a must. For other patients, chemo will do the heavy lifting of destroying cancer, so a stem cell transplant isn't necessary. I, however, was smack in the middle: A transplant could help me, but it could also hurt me. The decision was mine to make! I felt somewhat overwhelmed by this information and unsure of what to do. "Would you get the transplant if you were in my shoes?" I asked him. He dropped his head in thought to consider his answer.

> I was faced with a moment of truth and decision.

"Yeah," he said with a smile, "I'd do it—provided I'm the doctor." We both laughed yet realized it was a serious moment. My decision was relatively easy based on his response!

Dr. Fay informed me that I had a quirk in one of my chromosomes making the search for a perfect donor challenging. One part of my HLA typing was not common. I joked about my quirkiness and that this was not my only quirk, but at this moment, it was clearly the most important one for me; humor helped a lot while I was going through treatment. While I waited for a donor, I had four additional rounds of chemo—including another thirty-day hospital stay at Baylor and three rounds of outpatient chemo—to keep me in remission. As the days and months wore on, I wondered—and sometimes worried—if a donor would ever be found.

MY NEW BIRTHDAY

I remember the morning of May 12, 2006, like it was yesterday. The day was bright and sunny. I woke up early and prepared for the day ahead of me. I arrived at Baylor and adhered to the same low-key routine I had followed many times before at the infusion center. Yet there was something very different about the start of this day. The atmosphere was charged with an intensity I'd never felt before. I was fairly calm on the outside, but inside my heart was racing. I had waited eight long months for this day.

In the week preceding my stem cell transplant, I endured my fifth round of chemo to prepare my body for the donated stem cells. This was by far the most demanding chemo I had experienced. During the previous four rounds, I'd had side effects: an upset stomach, not wanting to eat, an aversion to certain smells, and periods of fatigue. But my experience was nothing like I'd heard about or expected. I was prepared (mentally) to be sick all the time, so I considered myself fortunate when I wasn't sick. Don't get me wrong, my experience was far from pleasant, but I knew others who went through a lot worse than I did.

The pre-transplant chemo was a different story. It was *tough*. I recall feeling awful from the moment the chemo started coursing through my body. My stomach was violently upset, and I vomited more than enough times to make up for my previously mild side effects. Needless to say, I was relieved when it was over.

When it was time for the transplant, an oncology nurse came into the room with what looked like a bag of yellow oatmeal and hung it on the IV pole next to my chair. She attached it to my central line, and for the next forty-five minutes, the stem cells slowly dripped through the IV into my body. Every now and then, a nurse would shake up the bag to keep it from clogging. When the last stem cell entered my body, I had a very surreal feeling. I couldn't put my finger on it, but I knew something very different was going on inside me. I had this vision of stem cells darting all over my body searching for a new home. The transplanted cells travel to the bone cavities and begin replacing old, damaged bone marrow almost immediately. In some extraordinary way, I actually felt this happening, and I wasn't just imagining it.

When the transplant process was done, several nurses came into the room and congratulated me by singing "Happy Birthday." May 12, 2006, would become my new birthday. A birthday I've celebrated every year since that day. I knew immediately that the transplant was my second chance at life. How many times, I wondered, do you get one of those? In that moment of great joy, I was immensely grateful to the anony-mous donor who selflessly made this second chance possible for me. That person made the momentous decision to make a difference in my life by giving me the opportunity to survive. This was a significant and unselfish gesture! I recognized the moment and was grateful beyond words!

> I had this vision of stem cells darting all over my body searching for a new home.

Every step of my journey with leukemia was a learning process, and at times the learning curve was extremely steep. Each new milestone in my progress presented new and unique challenges. I didn't have a game plan, and there certainly wasn't a cheat sheet to get me through every new stage. Now, hopefully on the road to recovery, there was only one goal ahead of me: to complete my fight with cancer and get back to normal. Little did I know that a few more challenges were headed my way.

CHAPTER 3

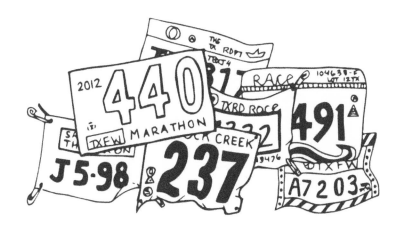

I Am a Survivor

"You can be a victim of cancer, or a survivor of cancer. It's a mindset."

—Dave Pelzer

A MAJOR SETBACK

For ten long months, I'd dreamed of being "normal" again. I didn't like being "the guy with leukemia." I just wanted to be me, Don Armstrong, and get back to life with the people for whom I cared. I can't tell you how many times other cancer patients have

told me the same thing. When I received my stem cell transplant,
I thought, "*This is it. I'm almost done.*" It was certainly true that the
transplant was a new milestone, but whether "normal" was right
around the corner or not was another question.

In fact, rather than nearing the finish line, I was just starting
another lap of my race. I had been told about GVHD—graft-versus-
host disease—prior to my transplant.
While I was aware that it was a possibility, I hadn't given it much thought.
GVHD can be a complication of an
allogeneic bone marrow transplant
from a donor who's not related to a
transplant recipient. The donor's bone marrow attacks the patient's
organs and tissues, impairing the tissues' ability to function and
increasing the patient's susceptibility to infection.

> In fact, rather than nearing the finish line, I was just starting another lap of my race.

Because I was so focused on the positives of the stem cell transplant, I really didn't pay much attention to the potential risks of
GVHD which Dr. Fay had described to me. True to form, I heard
what I wanted to hear. I didn't (or wouldn't) acknowledge the fact
that the GVHD could be worse than the leukemia itself, and that
the side effects of a transplant could take my life.

For the first thirty days after my transplant, I actually thought I had
evaded GVHD. That was, until I woke up one morning with what
appeared to be a rash on my arms and legs. It was the first, but hardly
the only, symptom of GVHD. Soon I also had almost uncontrolla-
bly itchy, dry skin. Ignoring the "twice daily" label recommendation

on the jar, I applied a steroid cream called Triamcinolone constantly, along with lotion. Then the dry mouth started. This wasn't your run-of-the-mill thirsty kind of dry mouth: It was in-the-desert-without-a-drop-to-drink dramatic movie-type thirst.

Next, I had difficulty swallowing, which made getting food and water down my throat almost impossible. For almost six weeks, I just couldn't swallow because it was so painful. I lost about thirty pounds during that time. At least I had that going for me! Ha! Plus, two to three times daily, I had to take my meds, which became a dreaded chore. I had to psych myself up to take them. On top of all of that, I developed severely dry eyes and painful mouth ulcers and sores.

Despite the physical reality of GVHD, the emotional impact was probably worse. I felt like I'd just come through a bad storm, only to face a hurricane. My dogged positivity and anticipation about the prospect of a "normal" future started to fail me. At times, it was tough to stay focused and have hope. I remember a particular evening I spent slumped over the kitchen sink with a mouthful of Gatorade that I could not swallow. I stared out the window, frustrated, before finally spitting the Gatorade into the sink. I savored the lingering taste in my mouth and asked myself, *"When is enough just enough?"*

To make a rough situation worse, my main caregiver, my wife, my rock through treatment, decided to leave me. She had been with me every second of every day from the moment my journey began and had been an instrumental part of my survival. One evening in mid-July, about sixty days after my transplant, she joined me in our living room to give me the news that she was moving out. Her decision took me completely by surprise. I wasn't prepared to handle this loss on top of everything else I was trying to overcome. I was devastated to say the least! I learned later from a social worker at Baylor that marriage is a common casualty among people dealing with long-term illness. It's a phenomenon known as "compassion fatigue," and it happens when caregivers give and give while receiving little in return. Eventually, they reach the bottom of their emotional reserves and simply break.

It was a lonely, confusing time, as I struggled to understand my wife's decision to leave, considering all we had been through together. On top of the emotional loss, without her financial support, I couldn't afford to remain in the three-bedroom house we shared, so I found a tiny, one-bedroom apartment in a nearby complex. I hadn't lived in an apartment in more than twenty-five years. To make matters worse, I was distraught to learn I would have to find a different home for my two beloved dogs because they couldn't live in the

> It was a lonely, confusing time, as I struggled to understand my wife's decision to leave, considering all we had been through together.

apartment with me. I initially tried to move myself because I didn't want anyone to know what I had been forced to do. For some reason unbeknownst to me, I selected an apartment on the third floor. Not a good decision. It didn't take me long to determine I was simply too weak from treatment to carry furniture and boxes up three flights of stairs. Thankfully, my son, David, offered to help me to move. Without his help, I couldn't have done it. David had been a quite source of comfort and support throughout my journey with cancer. He visited me every single day that I was at Harris. He didn't say a lot, but his presence was important and I somehow gained strength and courage from his visits.

At the same time that I was dealing with my GVHD symptoms and the collapse of my marriage, I was driving myself from Fort Worth to the infusion center at Baylor (Dallas) every morning, then driving to work another sixty miles to Cleburne for a new job. Following treatment, I was supposed to stay home in isolation so I could avoid potential infections from the outside world. The nurses would encourage me, on a daily basis, to go home, stay out of public areas with lots of people, and get plenty of rest. I thought they believed me when I told them I was going directly home. Little did I know they had heard my phone conversations offering directions to the crews who were working for me. Finally, one of them confronted me, "We know where you're going!" I was found out, but it was not in my nature to stay home and do nothing. Plus, I had to earn a living.

I hadn't worked since my cancer diagnosis and didn't really know what I was physically capable of doing, much less what my doctor would let me do. Perhaps more concerning, who would hire me knowing I was still going through treatment? Out of nowhere, I got a phone call from a family friend's son, Patrick Barley, whom I'd watched grow up and develop into a successful, young entrepreneur. He asked me if I had time to go with him

down to Cleburne, south of Fort Worth, to "look around." I didn't
know what that meant but couldn't really hide the fact that I
didn't have anything to do, so I said, "Sure! What's in Cleburne?"
"I'll show you," he told me.

We drove around Cleburne and then down to Rio Vista. Along
the way, he pointed out one gas drilling rig after another. I didn't
catch on to the significance of the conversation until Patrick told
me he'd started a natural gas pipeline construction company and
needed someone he could trust to oversee the field operations. I
was flattered, but I didn't know anything about the industry, and I
told him so. He wasn't concerned and
assured me I would get the hang of it.

> "It's like drinking
> water from a fire
> hydrant," he said. "It
> will almost drown
> you at first, until
> you start to figure
> out how to drink .
> . . and you will."

He knew I had a tremendous work
ethic and operated with attention to
detail. In addition, I had the project
management skills he was looking for
in a manager. "It's like drinking water
from a fire hydrant," he said. "It will
almost drown you at first, until you start to figure out how to drink
. . . and you will."

Believe it or not, this encouraged me because I knew he was
right. The fact that Patrick had enough confidence in me to give
me a chance was huge. It meant a lot to me. Plus, despite the daily
drives, a new job gave me something to look forward to every day.
This opportunity came along at just the right time.

Meanwhile, my symptoms continued. Maybe the most frustrating aspect of GVHD is that there's no set protocol for treatment. At least there wasn't ten years ago. The primary treatment objective is to find the right combination of drugs to reduce symptoms. At that time, I was taking at least three drugs specifically to control GVHD. The doctor's role is to eventually wean a patient off the drugs by gradually reducing the daily dosages. Of course, there's no set time-line since every patient's reaction to GVHD is different, so having any kind of realistic expectation is difficult.

At one point, Dr. Fay reduced my dosage because my symptoms seemed like they were under control. The new dosage worked for a few days, but then the symptoms returned. "Let's try this combination instead," he told me. "What do you mean, 'Let's try this?'" I asked. "Don't you *know* what will work? Isn't there some sort of plan?" "Not really," he said. "All I can do is react to your symptoms and come up with a different combination of drugs that hopefully works for you."

I admit this took a toll on me, wondering what, if anything, would ever address my symptoms. When it comes to GVHD, there is no one-size-fits-all treatment. Dr. Fay would try an approach, and if that didn't work, he simply tried something else. Nothing in the course of my illness had prepared me for the prospect of the symptoms of GVHD lingering. Still, even at the time, I knew I had to stay strong and hold onto my sense of determination, at least as much as I could, given the circumstances. There was no alternative. I couldn't give up. And unlike some GVHD patients, I was fortunate. Eventually, treatment did work—for good. I've been blessed to be off all medication for more than six years.

RECLAIMING NORMAL

Like many of you, I took normal for granted until it was taken away from me. I was coming off treatment for a life-threatening illness, which had ravaged my body in ways I didn't even fully understand. Still, I was eager to get back to the activities I enjoyed, such as running and working out in the gym. I had missed them during treatment. I asked Dr. Fay every day—every single day—following my stem cell transplant, "Can I start working out?" The answer was always an emphatic "NO!" He explained that my body had been through a great deal, and as a result, I just wasn't ready.

On September 12, 2006, I was given the okay to start working out, four months after my stem cell transplant. This was huge for me, since it was an opportunity to regain some *control* of my life—something cancer steals from every patient. This may seem like a small victory, but there are no words to describe my excitement when I got the green light. The small victories in my race meant so much and served to keep to me going in a positive direction. Dr. Fay told me, "Start slowly." He explained, "Your body will tell you what you can or can't do." Finally, I was taking care of myself without the medical profession's input. Now, I had the power to decide how to work toward improving my health.

> This was huge for me, since it was an opportunity to regain some control of my life—something cancer steals from every patient.

Two months into a regular workout routine, I started looking for a way to measure my improving strength and endurance. I woke up Thanksgiving

Day (2006) with nothing to do and a crazy notion to run the annual Fort Worth Turkey Trot, a 5K race. I am not sure where this idea came from, but I felt immediately committed. I figured it would be an excellent way to gauge my stamina. To my surprise, the race was much harder than I expected. However, I passed the test, not necessarily with flying colors, but I finished. More importantly, completing it inspired me to do more. Somewhere around the second mile of the 5K, I had a curious conversation with myself. *"Do you think you could run a marathon?"* I asked myself. I'm not sure where that thought came from or why I picked that that distance. However, my response was *"Yes! Why not a marathon?"* Outrageous maybe, but it was enough to motivate me toward yet another recovery milestone.

"Why not?" became my mantra. After all, why not train for and complete a marathon? There was no one to stop me, although I was compelled to ask for Dr. Fay's okay. Not surprisingly, he said "YES, go for it!" Conquering a 5K felt great, but was I ready for a bigger test of my stamina. I imagined how amazing it would feel to cross a finish line after 26.2 miles and quickly chose the 2007 Cowtown Marathon as my next endurance challenge. I didn't want the momentum of the moment to pass or come to an abrupt stop.

I started training the week after Thanksgiving. I gave myself approximately nine weeks to prepare. I really had no clue if that would be sufficient training time. I was, however, smart enough to ask for help from a local marathon guru who provided me with a schedule and some weekly feedback on my progress. I ran five or six days a week. Training was brutal on my body. It was like I had never run before. Every step I took, particularly in the beginning, was a challenge. I felt like my legs weighed a hundred pounds. Regardless, I was grateful to be training. Running quickly became my mental, emotional, and physical therapy.

On race day, I made it to the starting line confident that I would finish. That was my only goal! I had no true concept of pacing and had never trained more than fifteen miles or so.

> Running quickly became my mental, emotional, and physical therapy.

I had no sense of what miles 20 to 26.2 would be like physically or mentally, although I'd heard plenty about the dreaded "wall." My plan was simple: run as long and as far as I could and then walk the remainder of the distance. And that's exactly what I did. I ran for about sixteen miles and then walked to the finish line. And YES, I finished!

This marathon taught me a lot about myself. Not only was I on my way back to normal, I was starting to create a new normal, one that could be even more meaningful than my old one. It had taken a lot to reach the marathon finish line: illness, a glimpse of recovery, an unexpected setback, and a painful separation from my rock, my wife. Of all the places my journey could have taken me, it had led me here, to a place where I felt happy, healthy, and stronger than I'd been in a long time. Though I wouldn't wish what happened to me on anyone, I felt a strong sense of gratitude for the experience, and, more than that, for countless individuals—both known and unknown to me— who had made my recovery possible. I had no idea where to start, yet I wanted to pay it forward! I somehow, someway wanted make a difference in the lives of other people going through cancer.

TEAM IN TRAINING SHOWED ME THE WAY

In early 2007, I became aware of an organization called the Leukemia & Lymphoma Society (LLS). I checked out their website and was curious to learn more. The organization interested me because it funded blood cancer research and offered assistance to patients and their families. Soon after the Cowtown Marathon, I found myself back on the LLS website. I didn't really know what I was looking for, however, I knew I was searching for *something*. I read, with great interest, about LLS's Team in Training (TNT), a campaign that raises money for research while training individuals to complete an endurance event: marathon, triathlon, or cycling. I couldn't believe I could train for a marathon and raise money for blood cancer research at the same time. TNT was a perfect fit for me.

I went to a TNT information meeting to learn more. Within a week, I found myself at a kick-off event, where I felt an overwhelming feeling of appreciation for everyone in attendance. I quickly realized that everyone at this event showed up to selflessly commit themselves to fundraising and training. I immediately had a deep, emotional connection to the cause and its mission to fund a cure for blood cancer. I felt hopeful and excited. More than that, I knew I was in the right place. These were my people, and this was my purpose.

That night, I signed up for my first TNT event, the San Diego

Rock 'n' Roll Marathon. I trained with the Team, fundraised, and went to San Diego to complete the marathon. It was a life-changing, life-encouraging event for me and helped me embrace my "new normal" and move forward in the race of my life. I had no idea that so many people cared and were committed to finding a cure for blood cancer. Plus, I met so many amazing blood cancer survivors who had enthusiasm and zest for life. I was thrilled to be a part of something far greater than myself. I was beginning to realize I *could* make a difference. This was a turning point in my life.

Since March 2007, I have trained and raised money for nineteen additional TNT events, and I'm not done yet. My life, since my cancer diagnosis, has been enriched immensely because of TNT. In part, because I put on up my running shoes and run for an incredible cause. I've also found additional motivation to continue my life journey—my race—and recommit myself to live with purpose and gratitude each day. My experiences with this organization, first as a participant, then as a coach, an advocate, and now a Board of Trustee member, have changed me and hopefully others. I am still changing, and I'm determined to keep changing. My growth, I know now, will never end. To grow, you must be willing to change, even if what facilitates the change is a challenge you never anticipated encountering.

> To grow, you must be willing to change, even if what facilitates the change is a challenge you never anticipated encountering.

CHAPTER 4

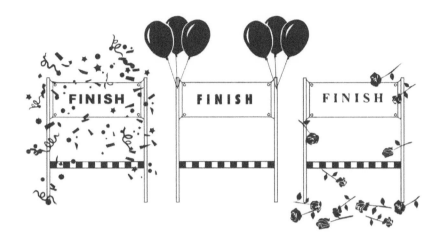

Identifying Your Race in Life

*"I have fought the good fight, I have finished
the race, I have kept the faith."*

—2 Timothy 4:7

In those difficult months following my stem cell transplant, running became my routine—and my therapy. I ran to be alone with myself, with nature, and with God. Running was when I did my greatest thinking and best soul searching. To this day, I always run in silence, with no music, to minimize distractions. However, my mind is anything but silent when I'm out pounding the pavement. In fact, almost every major decision I've made since 2006 was considered and confirmed on a run. Running is when I have my greatest clarity.

By mid-2009, I had remarried and was in good health. Things were going well. On a late-summer day, I was on an afternoon run with lots of time to think, when I realized that in a few short months it would be five years since my leukemia diagnosis. A five-year survivorship is a significant milestone for any cancer survivor. For AML survivors, it's a tremendous accomplishment. As I continued my run, it became clear to me that I needed to do something to celebrate. The farther I ran, the more excited I got.

When I arrived home, I could hardly contain myself and blurted out to my wife, "I'm coming up on my fifth year as a survivor. What can I do to celebrate?"

Immediately, I knew a celebration would involve running with TNT to raise awareness and money for LLS. With both excitement and urgency, I called my marathon coach, Jeanne Jones, to talk with her about my idea. I announced to her, "I know I want to run a marathon—more than one—but I don't know how many, when, or where. Do you think I'm physically ready to do something big?" I asked Jeanne.

"Definitely," she assured me confidently. "Let's figure out a way to make this happen!"

The next morning, I woke up with an idea. I would run ten marathons—five half and five full marathons—from January to December 2010. I wanted to do something big enough to get people to pay attention and say, "WOW!" Raising money and, more importantly, awareness about blood cancer would be the goals of this endeavor.

I puzzled over what to call my campaign, since "10 in 2010" was catchy but not significant. I had a lightbulb moment when I came across a Bible verse from 2 Timothy 4:7: "I have fought the good fight, I have finished the race, I have kept the faith." The scripture speaks about finishing the race and keeping the faith. The apostle Paul was looking back over thirty years of labor and work and was comparing his endeavors to an athlete who had been in a race and prevailed. I certainly

> 2 Timothy 4:7: "I have fought the good fight, I have finished the race, I have kept the faith."

could identify with Paul's sentiments, since I had fought my own fight with leukemia and had been victorious. Surely this was a metaphor that others could identify with as well. I knew instantly what to call my campaign: "Finish Your Race".

PUT YOUR RUNNING SHOES AWAY

As I mentioned in the introduction, I refer to my journey through life as a race. However, I want to get this out of the way right now, before going any further: Running isn't required to finish your race. You don't even have to like running. Heck, it's okay if you've never run a mile in your life. I'm not asking you to run an actual race.

However, I am asking you to open your eyes and heart and look inside yourself to clarify your own journey and how you can choose to be an agent of change. This is not something I probably would have done if not for my cancer diagnosis. It's incredible how your perspective can change when you learn your life may suddenly come to an end. Life is fragile and can change so quickly, with no warning. My battle with cancer allowed me to understand that everyone is traveling their own course, running their own race which is specific and unique to them.

Everyone's race is relatively short, since it's the length of your life. Everyone's race is also precious, which is just one more reason to make every day count. As you've probably learned by now, there are no guarantees in life. Your life is truly up to you. You have opportunities every day to define your outcome, your successes, your failures, and your value in this world. Recognizing and

> Life is fragile
> and can change
> so quickly, with
> no warning.

accepting these opportunities will help you take control of your race. Your decisions are your responsibility, and the results of your decisions are directly related to your choices. The decisions you make should be one of the most positive and rewarding things about your life and who you have become because *you* are in control of your success—yes, even your failure—and ultimately your own destiny. It's up to you!

If you are still unclear about what I mean by your "race," let me describe what your race is not. Life is not a foot race, road race, rat race, or horse race. It's not a competitive sport. Life shouldn't be about winning or losing. We are all winners, in our own way, based on our own definition of winning and how we run our own race!

You may sometimes feel driven to outdo others. You see what they have or do and you feel compelled, consciously or unconsciously, to keep up with the Joneses. Keep in mind, however, that trying to emulate those around you by striving for what they have may limit your potential. It is more important to just be yourself and know this is good enough.

Simply put, your race is your life's journey—your life in motion, progressing forward. Your race is who you are in the world, including your beliefs, priorities, motivations, and goals. It's not how you compare with someone else, but it is *how* and *who* you are in relation to your community, society, and ultimately the world.

> Your race is your life's journey—your life in motion, progressing forward.

I'm not here to prescribe a race for you. I can't do that! Only you can determine what your race is. You can't take someone else's journey, and they can't take yours. You have your own standards against which to judge your beliefs, priorities, motivations, and goals. Judging yourself against someone else's standards will only frustrate and discourage you, and it will repress your unique "you-ness." It's tough, I know, but strive to be the authentic you with no explanations or apologies.

Your race is the real deal, something you live every single day. It's the reason you get up every day—your **Why**. Your **Why** may be about money, personal satisfaction, recognition, achievement, giving, relationships, survival, or something else. It's likely a combination of all these things. Everyone has a **Why**. Have you ever sat down to consider yours, or, even better, have you written it down?

It took being diagnosed with leukemia, which created a new sense of urgency in my life, to sit down and discover my *Why*. But listen. You don't have to wait for that possibility; you have the chance to know your *Why* now. I wish I'd found mine prior to my diagnosis. When I did, my life transformed. With my *Why* (and my health), no matter what I did, I couldn't lose in life. Every day is a great day when you know what motivates you to get up in the morning, especially when you've had a close encounter with mortality.

UNDERSTANDING WHAT YOU WANT FROM YOUR RACE

In my life before cancer, my measure of success was based on how much money I made and how much "stuff" I could accumulate. My experience with cancer caused me to take a closer look at who I was, what motivated me, and what was important to me. As a result, I realized my priorities had been grossly out of focus. I had put work and financial success above the most important relationships in my life. The ten months I spent fighting for my life taught me that success—true success for me—is measured by more than financial gain. Financial success may be a part of your life, but it doesn't have to be the only thing in your life. Don't misunderstand me; there is nothing wrong with financial success—until financial success is all that fits into your day.

> Don't misunderstand me; there is nothing wrong with financial success—until financial success is all that fits into your day.

What do you want to accomplish in your life? It could be small or all-encompassing, local or global in nature. Let yourself think BIG. Are you striving for money, financial independence, achievement, recognition, status, power, or something else? Would accomplishing that ambition require you to become different than who you are today? Do you want to be different?

Your ambitions may feel daunting and out of reach, or they may inspire and motivate you. Are your ambitions compelling enough to make you take action? What would motivate you to accomplish your ambitions? Contentment, happiness, self-satisfaction, security, respect from others? All of these motivations are perfectly normal and acceptable. However, understand that these motivating factors can change over time, as my leukemia diagnosis changed mine.

When you think about your ambitions, how do they make you feel? Are you emotionally connected to them? Intellectually connected to them? Are your ambitions actually someone else's ambitions, maybe something you've seen a colleague or neighbor accomplish, or something someone else wants for you? Many times, children will follow their parents' dreams instead of their own, or a spouse will follow his or her spouse's *Why* instead of their own. Or perhaps you are living through someone else, through your significant other or your children's accomplishments.

It's not enough to identify your main ambition in life. It's not enough to simply know and understand your race. You need to know what's in it for you and the relationships around you. Have you considered the impact accomplishing your ambition will have on others? You need to understand how it affects your relationships and those around you. In other words, is accomplishing your ambition conducive to your personal or social well-being? Will it strengthen relationships with your family and loved ones? It's important that the people closest to you, including your spouse or significant other, family, and friends, know what gets you out of bed in the morning. Do your loved ones know and understand your *Why*? If not, make sure to communicate it to them. After all, no one can read your mind.

Prior to my cancer diagnosis, I wasn't very good at communicating to others what mattered to me. I kept almost everyone around me in the dark about what was important to me. Fortunately, this changed in the wake of my battle with cancer, as I began to understand the value and benefit of communication in all relationships. I am grateful for this new understanding and continue to grow and evolve almost every day.

What you strive to accomplish may very well make a difference in the lives around you, now and in the future. This is your legacy. It's worth taking some time now to ask what might at first seem like a morbid question to you: How do you want to be remembered? Carefully considering the answer may change the direction of your life and how you derive meaning from it. This was certainly the case for me.

If you feel that your past is holding you back, don't be concerned. You can use your past to your benefit. As Tony Robbins, American businessman, author, and philanthropist says, "The past does not equal the future," however, it can be a teacher. Learn from your past failures and use your past successes to motivate you. The past can be like a story you've finished. Instead of rereading it over and over, write a new one.

SO, WHAT IS YOUR RACE?

We all have a race in our life, even though you may not have given it much thought. Take a moment now to reflect on what matters most to you and what your priorities are in life. If you already have a pretty good idea of what drives you, great! You're a step ahead in the process. But if you are still unsure, don't worry. Keep reading. Maybe your priorities

> The past can be like a story you've finished. Instead of rereading it over and over, write a new one.

have changed recently or you've experienced some sort of setback. Know this: There is something major that moves you, even if you're not sure yet what that is right now.

I recently spoke with a man who asked me for career guidance. He had been in a business he loved early in his professional life. In his early thirties, he made a career change to make more money, switching to a totally unrelated career to which he devoted a decade of his life. Money became his driving force and for a while this was okay, until he realized he was unfulfilled and unhappy. He'd recently been dealt a professional setback and used this as an opportunity to look for a new direction. Since he had a wide variety of expertise, he decided to seek a number of different career options and see which one was the best fit. After listening to him for a few minutes, it was clear to me that, in his recent past, money had been his prime motivator. Finally, I asked him, "What do you really want to do? What's important to you? Are you trying to make as much money as possible, or do you want to be happy and fulfilled?" I got mixed answers to these questions, which told me he was unclear about his motivation and said, "Bottom line: Decide what you really want to do and focus on it. Don't be deterred by the obstacles in your way and be prepared for the ups and downs ahead. Go for what will provide fulfillment and makes you happy!"

I never heard back from this man, but his question regarding the choice of money or fulfillment is one I'm frequently asked. He knew the answer to his question; he simply wanted confirmation about what he already believed was best for him and his future. He was hoping, by talking with me, that I would verify his belief that he should pursue the profession which offered the most satisfaction for his professional life. When you are looking for a direction, the answer is quite often right in front of you. You simply need to be convinced.

> When you are looking for a direction, the answer is quite often right in front of you. You simply need to be convinced.

Knowing and understanding yourself is key to identifying what drives you. Finding your race is about self-discovery and requires an honest evaluation of yourself. Here are a few questions to get you started:

+ Do you have a purpose that burns inside of you, but you can't seem to act on it?

- When was the last time you thought about your life's purpose?
- Are you where you dreamed you'd be as a kid or young adult? Think back on what captivated your young mind when thinking about the future.
- Remember what you wanted to accomplish in your life.
- Do you feel trapped in a comfort zone that you don't believe you can escape?
- What do you dream about accomplishing, day and / or night?
- What motivates you on a day by day basis? Money, satisfaction, recognition, achievement, philanthropy, relationships, getting by, or something else?
- What fears, distractions, obligations, or other personal limitations do you feel are holding you back?

DON'T RUN YOUR RACE ALONE: THE IMPORTANCE OF RELATIONSHIPS

Though your race may be yours alone to travel, it's not all about you. In fact, it is seldom just about you. This understanding was an eye-opener for me. Before my cancer diagnosis, the thought that relationships should play a meaningful role in my life was a foreign concept to me. It is sad and disappointing for me to think back and realize how I failed to nurture the relationships in my life. It's even sadder that I had to experience such a major life event to change my thinking process. But, thanks to God, I saw the light.

Shortly after my stem cell transplant, a Baylor administrator asked me to visit with a group of rookie oncology nurses during their final orientation. As a cancer patient, I'd developed a special appreciation for this dedicated group of professionals. My role was to share my personal story of survival and describe the value I placed on the nurses who devoted so much time and effort to my well-being during treatment. I thought back to all the oncology nurses I'd met in the previous ten months. These nurses represented a key relationship for me during treatment and made such a difference in my recovery. They'd made an impact on my outlook, attitude, and overall health. The emotions I experienced during this orientation created an interest in me to understand what motivated these nurses to do their job. So I asked for permission to interview the nurses on the bone marrow transplant floor.

> Though your race may be yours alone to travel, it's not all about you.

I was fortunate to interview thirty-seven nurses and administrators, and the conversations were nothing short of eye-opening—especially when we talked about the role of relationships in their occupation. Almost every nurse explained how much they cherished and nurtured every relationship they had in the hospital, whether it was with a cancer patient, caregiver, doctor, or another nurse. They taught me the importance of paying attention, realizing everyone and every situation is vital and meaningful to the work they do, and that being open to hearing a patient's voice and emotions, no matter how difficult it was for them, was crucial for them.

"We listen with our hearts and not just our ears," one nurse told me.

I discovered that the way they handle relationships carries over to their relationships away from the hospital, with family and friends. Their experiences have taught them to care for and protect the relationships they have outside the BMT floor. One nurse explained to me, "Our work as oncology nurses serves as a daily reality check about our relationships and gives us great perspective for our own lives."

It was as if the relationship switch flipped to the "On" position in my head. I began to understand how imperative it is to cherish and nurture the relationships we have with family, friends, and, yes, even strangers. I realized the importance of striving (daily) to have a positive influence on others. In many ways, I had been solely focused on me without enough regard for those around me. I had been so zeroed in on succeeding and making money that I'd sacrificed essential time with loved ones to work long hours. I recognized I had missed the mark. It was a difficult reality to face; I had wasted time on the wrong priorities and goals for my life. Of course, my priorities since then have changed. These days, I'm deeply engaged in cultivating my relationships with others. What makes me get out of bed in the morning is the possibility of helping others find purpose and meaning in their lives. (We'll talk more about purpose in chapter 9.)

Understand this: You—yes, you—have the power to change someone's life. You aren't alone or isolated in your race. Think of the interactions you have with the people around you every single day. It is important to be mindful of these relationships, not just with friends and family, but also with neighbors, coworkers, and even strangers. *It's not just about what race you run, but the way you run it.*

You may not believe that you can influence other people's lives, but, make no mistake, you do. If you fail to share your thoughts, plans, dreams, and hopes with someone important to you or to listen to and help nurture theirs, you may miss out on something special. I know I did! If you take the low road when the high road seems harder to travel, you may have poor or negative consequences. In other words, don't try to win the day and make your point just to say or feel that you won. I know I did! None of us have all the answers. But here's what I've learned: None of us can go it alone.

> It's not just about what race you run, but the way you run it.

There was a time in my life when I thought I knew everything. I didn't ask for help because I didn't believe I needed help. In my greatest moment of vulnerability, I realized I needed a support system for the difficult times as well as the good times. In addition, I also needed to be a part of the support system for the people for whom I cared. Your relationships can provide you with guidance and encouragement, but you have to be open enough to them to give them a chance. Make no mistake, racing together will almost always have the most enduring and meaningful benefits for you and your loved ones.

YOUR CHOICE: FEAR OR COMMITMENT

Fear comes in many forms. Fear of failure can be overwhelming, while fear of success can lead to self-limitation and even self-sabotage. Fear of the unknown can cause intense anxiety. It takes us away from our feelings of safety and comfort. If you're feeling like fear is holding you back, you're not alone. I've been there right along with you many times. Here's the good news: Overcoming fear in order to make a change in your life is achievable, one step at a time. Meaningful change requires a persistent and consistent approach. It also requires unwavering courage. Above all, you must believe in yourself and believe that change is possible. A sincere commitment is required to make this happen.

When I think about fear, I am reminded of the famous quote from the 1933 inaugural address of our 32nd president, Franklin D. Roosevelt: "The only thing we have to fear is fear itself." FDR was so right. Fear holds people back every day. As simple as it might sound, fear can be a crippling emotion that stops even the toughest, strongest-willed person in their tracks. Don't let fear be the reason you don't do something.

> Overcoming fear in order to make a change in your life is achievable, one step at a time.

Acknowledging it, unpleasant though it may be, is the first step toward moving past fear.

I've learned a lot about fear as a marathon coach with Team in Training. "How can I possibly run or even walk a marathon?" first-timers often ask me. "I'm out of breath just walking from my car to the start line." TNT boasts that it will take participants from the couch to the finish line. Why? Because 85% of all new participants aren't athletic in any way, shape, or form when they begin. Many of them discover TNT when they are out of shape, unmotivated, and deeply in need of a change. Fear may have held them back, yet they still show up to give it a shot. "Becoming an endurance athlete takes time and effort," I tell them. "You're here, so you have some level of commitment already. Just take it one step at a time. I'm going to help you every step of the way." Small steps matter. Why? When I run a marathon, I never, ever think about the 26.2 miles ahead of me. Instead, I just put one foot in front of the other, and run a 5K ... and then I run another 5K and another. I break down what would otherwise be a terrifying distance into shorter, achievable sections knowing that if I combine them, I will eventually cross the finish line having gone 26.2 miles.

You can apply this same strategy to just about anything you attempt to achieve. Break down your ultimate achievement into smaller, more achievable segments. As you complete them one at a time, step by step, you draw closer to success until you've reached it. To chart it, or write it down, makes it even more believable in your mind and serves as a visible reminder of your success.

> If you allow yourself to believe you can, you awaken the ability within yourself to succeed.

As a coach, my role is to ease trainees' minds, to give them a doable plan, and to reassure them step by step, mile by mile, that they will get to the start line, and, ultimately, they'll finish their race. If you allow yourself to believe you can, you awaken the ability within yourself to succeed. This method has led to some dramatic, emotional moments as teammates cross a finish line that months earlier seemed impossibly far away. I've shared tears of joy with dozens of these successful finishers.

About seven years ago, a new participant who was overweight and out of shape joined the Team. He lacked the confidence to believe it was even possible to complete an endurance event, but to his credit he had enough conviction to show up on the first day of training and every week for the entire season. He did not let fear stop him. Over the course of the season, he lost almost seventy-five pounds, got in shape (physically and emotionally), and finished a half marathon. The feeling of success, of overcoming a huge, stop-in-your-tracks fear, was so inspiring for him that he went on to complete numerous marathons and ultramarathons (any distance longer than 26.2 miles). Many TNT participants who thought they could never train for a marathon not only finish their first event, they decide to keep racing—because now they know they can!

All successful finishers, in TNT and in life, share a number of traits in common: They recognize their fear, believe change is possible, commit to change, and implement a plan for change, one step at a time. They don't allow their lack of progress to discourage or overwhelm them. They just keep pressing ahead, step by step by step.

The next eight chapters are designed to empower you to run faster, harder, and better so that you can reach your goals long before you believed possible. My battle with cancer was my catalyst to take my race more seriously. Hopefully, you won't need such a traumatic event to motivate you to make changes. It's true what they say: Life is short. So don't wait—take charge and take action. Life's trauma and drama won't transform you until you take action to change yourself. It's up to you to take control of your life, because no one else can or will do it for you. *Finish YOUR Race* is about starting and not giving up, no matter what.

Ready to forge ahead? Let's get started!

CHAPTER 5

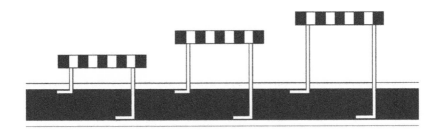

Adversity Happens: Jumping Over Hurdles

"It's not what happens to you, but how you react to it that matters."

—Epictetus

Do you enjoy riding roller coasters? Do you remember how you felt the first time you rode one? Or how you felt *before* you rode it, while you were anxiously waiting in line? Once you got in, the attendant tightened a strap around your waist as you prepared to take off. You can't get out. You *had* to take the ride. Then you suddenly started to move forward. Remember that lurch forward as you approached that first steep hill ahead of you? As you climbed, the *clack, clack, clack* of the tracks got louder, and you had no clue what awaited you at the top.

Well, that's exactly what I experienced on that first day in the hospital preparing for my initial round of chemo—and in the weeks that followed. Three or four days into the first chemo, I was on the downhill part of the ride. The ride down is much better than the ride up because at least you have a better idea of where you're headed. The tracks may twist and turn—you may even turn upside down—but you are feeling more confident that you'll survive the ride in one piece.

The ride wasn't always enjoyable. However, after the first big hill, my first round of chemo, I felt okay because I had a better understanding of what to expect. I had five total rounds of chemo, but the first round set the tone for the other four. Because I knew what was coming, I was able to confront my fears, and with each progressive round of chemo, it got easier to raise my hands above my head as I climbed to the top of more hills and sped down the other side.

I used this roller-coaster story at an LLS School and Youth assembly back in 2009. This was a day of celebration for a thirteen-year-old student who had survived leukemia. Her classmates supported their brave friend throughout her journey with cancer. I was struggling to find a way to describe my experience with leukemia in a way that these students could relate to. It's a story I still use because it so accurately describes my uncertainty about my diagnosis and how

I overcame it. It describes the approach we can all take when confronted with adversity: Recognize the challenge, confront it, and overcome it.

It also illustrates how adversity can impact your life in a positive way and help you grow. We usually associate adversity only with negative outcomes,

> Recognize the challenge, confront it, and overcome it.

with what is going wrong, and yet my battle with leukemia has led me to so many positives in my life. My diagnosis had the potential for tragic results, but ultimately it became a major turning point in my life—for the better. Know that you, too, can be dealt a crazy hand in life and still turn it around for the better.

WHEN THE GOING INEVITABLY GETS TOUGH

Adversity is an inevitable part of everyone's life. It's certainly not something we plan our lives around. However, if we're realistic, we know it's not a matter of "if" but "when" it will affect our lives. Even so, tragedy, misfortune, illness, and setbacks usually come as surprises, often when we least expect them, typically without warning.

Accepting that adversity is a fact of life and learning how to transform it into a positive motivator can be challenging. Just the possibility of adversity can dictate your daily decisions, paralyze you, or limit your expectations—but it shouldn't. Don't allow the specter of adversity to influence how you live your life.

For some people, encountering adversity means leaping to a worst-case scenario, one in which we are powerless to act. But it doesn't have to be that way. You certainly can't plan for it, but you can choose to not let it consume you. Adversity, and more importantly overcoming it, can be a blessing and lead to better things in your life. It was for me! As strange as this might sound, leukemia changed almost every aspect of my life for the better. It's inevitable that at some point, life *will* knock you down, but you must get up each and every time and move forward. Deciding—now—how to handle unexpected setbacks when they happen will help you feel stronger and more determined to overcome them.

> Adversity, and more importantly overcoming it, can be a blessing and lead to better things in your life.

WHAT YOU CAN AND CAN'T PLAN FOR

Everyone experiences stumbling blocks from time to time— rush-hour traffic, a minor fender bender, an appliance breaking, a lost wallet, a child coming down with a cold, and more. But as life progresses, sometimes more serious hardships can really rock our world. For me, the unexpected adversity of a life-threatening illness stopped me in my tracks. Everything in my world was put on hold. You may have experienced something similar recently, such as the death of a loved one, a job loss, the breakup of a relationship, or a natural disaster which put your life on pause.

In my battle with cancer, I learned a hard lesson: Adversity has its own timetable. My leukemia diagnosis didn't come with a forecast of what would happen each day. From the first day of my fight against leukemia, I never quite knew what to expect. The time frame of my illness and recovery was uncertain, and there was no script to follow. I craved and expected more certainty in my treatment and its outcome, but seldom found it to happen in a clear and predictable manner.

As human nature would have it, even early on, I heard only what I wanted to hear. As I understood it from my doctor, I would be in the hospital for about a week. When I later asked one of my nurses to confirm this, she replied, "Oh no, you can expect to be in the hospital for at least thirty days. We really get to know our AML patients well because of the length of their hospital stay." How did I miss this message in my doctor's comments to me? Wishful thinking and selective hearing, I'm sure.

From the outset of my treatment, I always latched onto the best-case scenario for my treatment and never really chose to believe in a less-than-positive outcome. One round of chemo became two, three, four, five rounds, and then, after all that was complete, a quirk in my chromosome made finding a stem cell donor difficult. My hope for finding a donor quickly turned into an eight-month search. I wondered, and sometimes worried, whether a donor match would ever be found. Still, I refused to give up. Even after my stem cell transplant, my recovery took another detour, through GVHD. Over and over again, I realized that hardship is nothing if not unpredictable. You can't plan for it, but you can persevere.

MENTAL TOUGHNESS

As an endurance athlete, I am keenly aware that mental toughness is crucial to completing a half marathon, marathon, triathlon, or a one hundred-mile cycle ride. Mental toughness means pushing ahead through difficult circumstances with confidence. It's doing what needs to be done in spite of obstacles. I believe we all have the mental-toughness trait within us, and when the circumstance calls for it, we are ready, willing, and able to use it.

> Mental toughness means pushing ahead through difficult circumstances with confidence.

No matter how many races I've run, no matter how well I've trained, no matter how good the weather is on race day, I know there will be a least one moment of pain at some point in the race. I can't tell you when or where, I can only tell you it *will* happen, and when it does, I might be tempted to think I can't go on and should stop. It's predictable for me to want to quit at least three or four times during a marathon, and so I've become mentally prepared for that moment to arrive. When it does, I'm ready. My strategy for pushing through may be as simple as saying to myself, "Trust your training!" All it takes is a little positive self-talk to get over the hurdle of doubt and keep on keeping on.

Mental toughness works for me in endurance races, and I know it will work for you when you encounter adversity. You can't predict adversity, but you can prepare yourself mentally for the inevitability that it will find you. Don't trick yourself into thinking life will always be footloose and fancy free. Accept now that adversity will play a role in your life, and learn to trust that you can handle whatever comes your way.

Knowing that adversity is something you will encounter puts you in a position of strength. Realizing that there are a few things you should *not* do when you reach one of life's inevitable impasses puts you in position to begin to overcome the adversity quickly and appropriately. Don't take unnecessary risks, reach for unrealistic solutions, and, most importantly, don't overreact. Attitude plays a huge role in overcoming hardship, as you will see in the next chapter. So, think positive! No matter what life throws at you, you always have the opportunity to decide for yourself how to face the unexpected. The more mentally prepared for adversity you are, the better equipped you'll be to take action.

Because everything moved very quickly when I was diagnosed with leukemia, I didn't have much time to think about the seriousness of the illness. I realized early on, however, that I was fighting for my life. Instinct overrode everything in my head and heart with one singular goal: Survival. Until that point, life had thrown me plenty of curveballs to keep me on my toes. Certainly, none of them were as serious as leukemia, but by the time I went in for my first chemo treatment, I had plenty of experience with the unexpected. Dealing with these setbacks helped me to be mentally prepared—mentally tough—when cancer came knocking.

During the 2007–2009 economic decline, I learned that overcoming one hardship is no guarantee that you won't face another.

As I mentioned in an earlier chapter, I landed a job in the oil and gas business in early 2006. It was a much-needed source of income for me during a time when both my health and financial future felt precarious. Oil and gas, at least, would always be a sure thing—or so I thought. In my mind, my job in the Barnett Shale was secure . . . until an economic downturn resulted in a dramatic drop in the price of natural gas. Almost immediately, jobs dried up, and I was laid off for the first and only time in my life.

Being laid off was a real double whammy. After temporarily losing my ability to work due to leukemia, my job in the pipeline business was a lifeline that helped me reclaim some much-needed financial stability. I was just starting to dig my way out of a financial hole when the bottom dropped out of the industry, and my job was terminated. I was facing a huge and very different challenge for the second time in less than three years. It was a brutal blow, but thankfully my mental toughness immediately kicked into overdrive. I had a plan and was ready to take action. I'd updated my resume on a regular basis, so I didn't need to do much to have it ready. I had continued to maintain professional relationships in my primary area of expertise, the golf business, so I had a strong network. I was quick to call everyone I knew to let them know I was looking for a new job and set up meetings with prospective employees. Being laid off was actually a blessing in disguise, as I found my way back to the golf business—a business I still loved and do to this very day.

The Great Recession of late 2007 to mid-2009 impacted millions of people. Maybe you were one of them. During this time, thousands of people lost their homes, their jobs, or both. Many of these folks were ill prepared for the unexpected. They had no plan in place for adversity. They felt paralyzed. Among my friends, some refused to accept that they needed, urgently, to take action. Embarrassed and in denial, some withdrew from their social circles. Instead of updating their resume and reaching into their professional network, some friends seemed stuck in a mentality of loss and negativity. As you can imagine, many of these friends found themselves unemployed for much longer than those friends who had prepared for the possibility of the unexpected.

Like most of us, you've probably hit a few bumps along your life's journey. Let them be instructive to you. As much as possible, prepare yourself emotionally, mentally, physically, and spiritually for adversity. Have a plan of action to be ready for adversity. Mental toughness will be a factor in overcoming adversities of all types.

HOW DO YOU REACT TO ADVERSITY?

There are four ways to react to adversity. You can:

1. Allow it to define you
2. Allow it to consume and ultimately destroy you
3. Allow it to strengthen you
4. Allow it to be an opportunity for change and growth

Though it may not feel like it sometimes, hear me clearly: The choice is *yours*.

This was key among those invaluable insights I gained from

interviewing the Baylor oncology nurses. Because they're confronted with adversity every day at work, certainly more hardship than the average person, they've refined their approach to life's difficulties. They choose to look at each patient as a special individual, and they recognize that each person's reaction to difficult circumstances is unique. This thought or type of thinking influenced how they approached their work and, ultimately, life. As one nurse explained to me, "We don't let the small things in life bother us." Instead, they find a way to transform challenges into positive experiences and opportunities for growth. They certainly don't take life for granted. They work in a setting where the people they care for sometimes die, so they understand the value of life and fervently embrace it. One nurse asked me, "If you were to live your life thinking something unexpected and tragic might happen tomorrow, would you live differently today?" For all of us, I believe the answer would be a resounding YES!

> One nurse asked me, "If you were to live your life thinking something unexpected and tragic might happen tomorrow, would you live differently today?"

Intellectually, we understand that unexpected difficulties will happen from time to time. However, we can't let these difficulties define us. We have a choice to react consciously and intentionally. As William Arthur Ward, one of America's most quoted writers of inspirational maxims, said, "Adversity causes some men to break, others to break records."

THE ACTION-REACTION CONNECTION

As I've already mentioned, your reaction to adversity is more important than the hardship itself. Your reaction shapes your character and sets the tone for how you'll overcome setbacks—or not. The next time you face a challenge—even a minor one, like traffic—try to take a step back and observe your reaction. Do you become immediately frustrated? Does your mind immediately leap to the worst-case scenario—being late for a dinner reservation or missing an important meeting? Do you become angry at other drivers? Or are you able to take a level-headed, logical approach, maybe calling your dinner companion or colleagues to let them know that, though it's not certain, there's a possibility you might be late?

Early in my battle with leukemia, I had to figure out how to deal with my illness. I instinctively knew that I couldn't let it define me as a person, and that my reaction to this adversity would determine my character and affect my future. I made a conscious, instinctive decision. I didn't have to think about having a positive mindset when my treatment started. It just happened! In other words, I knew adversity was a possibility. I didn't know when or to what degree. I certainly had no idea of the potential severity. However, mentally, I was prepared. Though I'm talking about my illness, the same technique or mindset will help with almost any adversity you are facing, from losing a job, a relationship ending, the death of a loved one, or other life events.

Once it was clear that I would be stuck on the seventh floor at Harris (during my first round of chemo) for at least a month, I made the decision to maintain as much normalcy as possible. To make this happen, I needed structure and routine, just like I had at work and home. I did everything I could to stick to a daily pattern. I didn't want to be in the hospital, so I chose to act as if I wasn't in the hospital. I never wore a hospital gown. Every morning, I got up about 6:00 and shaved, showered, and dressed. My outfit for the day was a pair of shorts and a collared golf shirt. I ate breakfast, when I was up to it, and waited for my doctor to come by for our morning conversation. The remainder of the day was devoted to reading or visiting with friends. I refused to watch television during the day so I didn't turn it on until the evening news. As the effects of the chemo took a toll on my body, I would occasionally nap out of necessity because I just couldn't stay awake.

I also chose to stay active, rather than thinking of myself as sick or helpless. My first priority was physical activity, so I made a commitment to stay as fit as possible. Every afternoon or evening, I would walk the hallways for my daily exercise. The idea of walking the hallways may sound strange, I know, but for me it was invigorating. At first, I could only walk for fifteen minutes, but I soon built up to an hour. My son brought me weights, so I could add weight lifting to my routine. This sense of normalcy helped me deal with the realities of my diagnosis and treatment, since I couldn't leave the floor, and I couldn't leave my room without a mask on. It was important for me to make the best of each day, insofar as I could choose to do so. Even if I couldn't control the cancer, I knew I was in control of my reaction to my diagnosis and treatment.

The Greek philosopher Herodotus said, "Adversity has the effect of drawing out strength and qualities of a man that would have lain dormant or absent." Truer words were never spoken. The setbacks you'll encounter in your life have the potential to lead to personal growth. They certainly did for me. Overcoming adversity can give you momentum and confidence in your life. If you control your reaction to adversity, adversity won't control you.

> The setbacks you'll encounter in your life have the potential to lead to personal growth.

DEALING WITH ADVERSITY

When an unexpected misfortune comes crashing into your world, what can you do? Here are some strategies that have worked for me:

- Stay calm. When in doubt, take a deep breath.
- Remain grounded. Avoid jumping to a worst-case scenario or overreacting.
- Trust yourself and your instincts. You're stronger than you think.
- React with clear and rational thinking by defining your options and thinking through solutions.
- Find ways to maintain a sense of normalcy, even if it's as simple as committing to brush your teeth each morning and evening. Or, in my situation, declining to wear a hospital gown.
- Focus and do your best to avoid being swept up by anxiety or fear.

- Believe in yourself and trust in your faith for courage and strength.

- Seek support from family, friends, a mentor, a professional counselor, or a minister.

- Develop an achievable game plan and have a backup plan in the event that your primary approach doesn't give you the results you need.

- Sleep on it. The older I've gotten, the more I understand that it's better to think before you react to just about anything. Time will assist you in clarifying your plan.

- Understand that no matter what, nothing and no one can prevent you from choosing how to react to a challenge.

- Never, ever quit—adversity is your call to action. So take action. Remember, even not taking action is a decision.

THE OTHER SIDE

During treatment, my cancer had control of my life. Following treatment, I demanded to be back in control, and it was up to me to make this happen. There was nothing easy or quick about the process of recovery. As I learned, it takes time, patience, and more time. Still, because I recognized that I had a choice about how to deal with my illness, I emerged, after a long recovery, stronger, wiser, and more resilient.

> You don't have to have a life-threatening disease to experience a life-changing challenge.

You don't have to have a life-threatening disease to experience a life-changing challenge. There's no better time than right now to prepare for the possibility that life will throw you a curveball, and if you're facing one of those hurdles right now, read on. The next chapters describe specific strategies that will help you approach any challenge with more clarity and focus, as well as offer some real-world solutions to help you finish your race.

CHAPTER 6

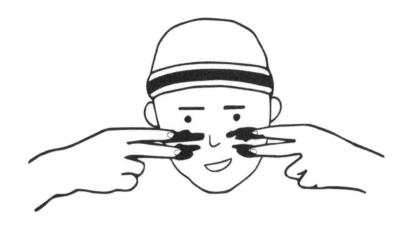

Attitude Is Everything: Developing a Winning Attitude

"Nothing can stop the man with the right mental attitude from achieving his goal."

—Thomas Jefferson

Like almost everyone, my attitude has been tested on more than one occasion. No matter the challenge, I've always tried to carry on with a positive mental attitude. I read minister and author, Norman Vincent Peale's book *The Power of Positive Thinking* when I was in my early teens, and it made a tremendous impression on me. I recommend it for anyone looking for principles on positive thinking. The biggest takeaway from the book for me was that what you think can impact who you are. I also learned that what you believe can determine your outcome. As a result, I've long since adopted a glass-half-full outlook, and this approach served me well during my battle with cancer. Though we might often hear that attitude matters, what I went through revealed in the most serious way the power of a *positive* attitude.

The power of attitude didn't even register with me until I had an insightful conversation with Dr. Fay late in my treatment. He was describing my progress and trying to explain the reasons for my success beyond medical treatment. Much to my surprise, Dr. Fay told me, "Your attitude made a significant difference in your recovery. I wish that you could speak to some of my other patients to share the value and benefit of a positive outlook." I didn't really know what to say. I'd never thought about my attitude as a game changer. The way I approached my situation felt comfortable, even normal. This might sound odd, but I don't think it even occurred to me, before that conversation, that everyone didn't react with a positive attitude given a similar circumstance. For me, this came naturally.

THE ORIGINS OF ATTITUDE

Your attitude characterizes the way you respond and relate to people, circumstances, and situations. You might not even be aware of it sometimes, but your attitude is constantly influencing the way you perceive your world and interact with it. Attitude comes from within and is the accumulation of learned beliefs, values, and assumptions. The accumulation process starts at a very young age and is usually influenced first and foremost by our parents. As we grow and mature, our life experiences continue to influence and shape our attitudes. Attitudes may reside in our subconscious mind, but they play an even more important role in our conscious decisions and behaviors.

Contrary to what you might think, attitude is not an emotion or feeling. It's an outward behavior, an active rather than passive process. It's a decision you make regarding how you handle anger, fear, sadness, joy, love, or surprise. In other words, if something happens to you or around you, your reaction is based on the sum total of your life experiences. Attitude is not **what** you think, but **how** you think.

> Attitude is not what you think, but how you think.

Keep in mind, no single reaction determines your attitude. Your attitude is the accumulation of your reactions.

As a young man learning to play golf, I wasn't sure if I had the talent to really excel at the sport, but I was learning more about the game every day that I practiced and played. Some days I played better than others. Invariably, during a round of golf, I made a few bad shots, which influenced my view toward the game. Fortunately, I made many more good shots, which encouraged me to keep going. If I had chosen to focus on the poor shots, I may have decided to quit. Instead, I allowed the good shots to motivate me to continue playing while honing my golf skills.

But attitude isn't just outfacing: how you perceive the world. Your attitude impacts the way others react to you. As an author and motivational speaker Keith Harrell wrote, "Attitude is everything. It governs the way you perceive the world and the way the world perceives you." It might not feel like it sometimes, but your attitude is transparent. Whether you're positive, negative, pessimistic, optimistic, or apathetic, your attitude reveals your relationship to your self-esteem, self-acceptance, and self-affirmation.

> My attitude meant, quite literally, the difference between living and dying.

And here's something else you should you know about attitude: It can 100% determine the course of your future. And that's something to seriously think about. My attitude meant, quite literally, the difference between living and dying. It's *that* important.

ATTITUDE CAN CHANGE YOUR OUTCOME

My junior year in high school, I was on the golf team representing the Robinson Rams, in Fairfax, Virginia. We were talented enough to win the district and regional tournaments, which qualified us for the high school state golf tournament. Only four of us were eligible to go to the state tournament. I was one of the four. We had all worked hard and were confident we would win the tournament handily.

A week before the state high school tournament, I decided to join a pickup basketball game. I liked to play basketball, but I wasn't really very good. Nonetheless, I joined in when a team needed another player. Someone passed the ball to me, and I went up for a jump shot. I made the shot, but when I landed, I heard a pop and felt instant throbbing pain in my right ankle. I laid on the ground in agony with only one thought in my head: "*The state golf tournament is next week.*"

Needless to say, Coach Howard was not very happy with me. Neither were my teammates, but they rallied, encouraging me that I'd recover quickly. Here's the good news: Nothing was broken in my ankle. I did, however, have a severe sprain which made it difficult to walk for the first few days. Still, I decided early on that I was going to play in the golf tournament. I'd practiced long and hard to qualify for this golf tournament, and nothing was going to deter me.

My ankle did improve in the week leading up to the golf tournament. The morning of the first round, a coach from another team offered to tape my ankle. This provided me with additional stability, although I still had trouble pushing off my right ankle to finish the swing. Nonetheless, I played with a can-do attitude. I hit one shot at a time and played one hole at a time. It wasn't my greatest round, but I played and was absolutely thrilled. I finished with a first round 80 and a second round 77. Not my best, but respectable. Our team finished third overall, which was a victory for us considering my injury.

The moment I heard that horrible pop, I could have given up and resigned myself to my injury. I could have stayed home with an ice pack on my ankle feeling sorry for myself. Instead, I tapped into my mental toughness and pushed through the pain. I probably had no business playing in that tournament, but I was determined. My positive attitude kept me in the game and propelled me to finish. Attitude changed the outcome.

Think about it for a moment. Could your attitude, good or bad, make an impact on the outcome of a specific event in your life? Let's say you're vying for a job you really want. You could choose to pursue it with a positive outlook, or you could take a casual, "Whatever, I don't stand a chance of being hired" mentality. Both attitudes will impact your outcome, but only one will help you get what you want. The beauty of attitude is you can apply a positive approach to almost any area of your life. You will quickly understand that attitude is essential to receiving your desired outcome. Like it or not, your attitude has affected or will affect nearly every outcome of your life—past, present, and future. It affects your relationships with family and friends and impacts how others see you. It plays a role in your career and, yes, even your health.

Make no mistake: In many ways, attitude can be the make-or-break element in your life. Your attitude can lead you to a solution, or it can compound your problems and make them worse, so make sure you are conscious of your attitude.

ATTITUDE IMPACTS EVERYTHING AROUND YOU

John Maxwell, author, speaker, and pastor said, "People may hear your words, but they feel your attitude." Positive or negative, good or bad, encouraging or discouraging, people sense your attitude and often react to it. Think about a time in your life when someone else's attitude affected your own, for better or worse. How did their outlook change your feelings about a situation or that person? More than likely, someone else's attitude has, at least once, affected your attitude.

> Your attitude can lead you to a solution, or it can compound your problems and make them worse, so make sure you are conscious of your attitude.

Remember, your attitude is the result of years of life experiences. We know that attitudes can be infectious. Whether someone has a positive or negative attitude impacts the tenor of your mental reaction and behavior: in other words, your attitude. We get excited and enthusiastic in response to someone's upbeat and positive attitude. We can also become indifferent and turned off by someone's pessimistic or negative attitude. As a result, be aware that your attitude can affect others and ultimately the circumstances around you. It's never too late to be mindful of your attitude. This should be an internal, automatic process that happens without any conscious thought or awareness, but this isn't always the case. Therefore, make the process of identifying or recognizing your attitude a situation by situation acknowledgement of how you react, respond, or behave to a circumstance or person.

Think about it. What does your attitude convey? Your attitude can tell a story and paint a picture for others. Your attitude offers a glimpse into the way you think. My reaction to a diagnosis of leukemia was to stay upbeat and in the moment, as much as possible, but this isn't the case for everyone. As I've met other blood cancer patients over the years, I've been struck by the scope of their emotional reactions to their diagnosis. Some people were consumed by their diagnosis and were only able to focus on the possible negative aspects of the disease. But other people took their illness in stride and made the best of every single day. We may not all be programmed to be positive from an early age. This depends on the models we had growing up, but if your default mode is seeing the glass half-empty rather than half-full, it might very well be because someone in your life taught you, probably by example, to see it that way. There's nothing essentially right or wrong with either approach, however, keep in mind, your attitude does impact the outcome. You *can* change it, and as Dr. Fay confirmed, your attitude, like your approach to any circumstance or situation, can be the determining factor in overcoming a serious situation.

So ask yourself, what impact does your attitude have on others? Is your attitude consistent, constant, stable, or always changing as the circumstances vary, similar to the waves in the ocean, up and down? Do you like what your attitude represents about you to others? Are you satisfied with your attitude? Is your attitude leading you in your desired direction? Is your attitude positive enough to move you forward? If someone wrote your eulogy, what would they say about you? Do people seek you out when they need support? What do you contribute to a conversation when someone is having a tough time? Are you a person others seek out to raise their spirits? It shouldn't take you long to find or determine the answers to these questions. It's worth the effort to consider all of them. In addition, ask a trusted friend for an assessment of your attitude. Is their assessment similar to yours? Hang on for the answer—you may be surprised!

YOU ARE IN CONTROL OF YOUR ATTITUDE

My battle with cancer taught me a great deal about myself and others. One of the most significant lessons was accepting that attitude is a choice. Like me, you always have a decision—a choice—to make. I could have resigned myself to the negative possibilities of my diagnosis, but it wasn't in my nature to do so. Instead, I chose to remain upbeat and positive. My attitude was up to me and no one else. No matter how sick I was, no one could take that choice away from me.

> One of the most significant lessons was accepting that attitude is a choice.

In times of adversity, even if everything feels out of your control, understand that you do have control of your reaction. It's your choice. You make choices about your attitude from the moment you wake up in the morning until your head hits the pillow at night. You are reacting to various circumstances every single hour of every single day of every single week, month, and year of your life. At any point, at any time, you have the opportunity to define your attitude and change it, if it's not serving you in a positive way. You are the only one responsible for your attitude. You own the impact of your attitude in your life. Understand and be aware that external circumstances and other people are not honest excuses for a negative attitude.

I have experienced firsthand the attitude of newly diagnosed cancer patients. Since my recovery, I've had the opportunity on numerous occasions to visit with patients to offer support and perspective. I remember walking into one patient's hospital room and being astonished by the homey appearance. It felt like I was walking into this woman's living room. I asked her about the changes to the room. Her response was unexpected but reflected her positive attitude. With a broad, beaming smile, she explained, "I understand I will be here for at least a month. As a result, I decided to make this room a reflection of my home." Following a terrific conversation, I left with a happy heart and a lot of hope for this amazing woman who was facing incredible adversity.

The very same week, I walked into another patient's room and was greeted with a gloomy scene. The room was dark and cold. The blinds on the windows were closed, and there was only one faint lamp shining. My conversation with the patient was negative and halting, with little hope for a positive outcome. I asked him how he was handling his situation. His response was unexpected but not unheard of, considering his circumstances: "I don't want to die," he said. I did my best to offer a positive outlook, as he pointed to a small framed picture of a little girl. He explained with tears in his eyes that the girl was his daughter. There wasn't much I could say in that moment to lift his spirits or encourage him. I did my best, however, by the end of the visit, I left feeling deflated and anxious for the journey he faced ahead.

These were two individuals with similar diagnoses but very different attitudes. I understand both patients' perspective and respect both attitudes. Believe me, I get it. Cancer is tough. However, in my heart, I couldn't help but hope for a more positive attitude for the male patient. Unfortunately, I wasn't able to influence his outlook, yet I prayed that over time he would find a positive attitude to lift his spirits.

You can't control all the events of your life; however, you can control your attitude. You have the power to be positive or negative. Choosing to be positive leads to self-encouragement, self-motivation, and excitement about

> You can't control all the events of your life; however, you can control your attitude.

life. Choosing to be negative can lead to self-defeat, self-pity, and self-doubt. The outcome of your life is about your attitude and the choices you have made, are making, and will make in the future. You are in control.

Chuck Swindoll, pastor and author, sums up my thoughts about the control we have over our attitude with these insightful words:

Attitudes

The longer I live, the more I realize the importance
of choosing the right attitude in life.
Attitude is more important than facts.
It is more important than your past;
more important than your education or financial situation;
more important than your circumstances, your successes, or your failures;
more important than what other people think, say or do.
It is more important than your appearance, your giftedness, or your skills.
It will make or break a company. It will cause a church to soar or sink.
It will make the difference between a happy home or a miserable home.
You have a choice each day regarding the attitude you will embrace.

Life is like a violin.
You can focus on the broken strings that dangle,
or you can play your life's melody on the one that remains.

You cannot change the years that have passed,
nor can you change the daily tick of the clock.
You cannot change the pace of your march toward your death.
You cannot change the decisions or the reactions of other people.
And you certainly cannot change the inevitable.
Those are the strings that dangle!
What you can do is play on the one string that remains – your attitude.
I am convinced that life is 10 percent what happens to me
and 90 percent how I react to it.
The same is true for you.

Chuck Swindoll

The remarkable thing about Mr. Swindoll's message is we do have a choice every day regarding the attitude we embrace for that day. We are solely in charge of our attitudes. Every single day, your attitude is up to you. These are words you can apply to your life: Now!

SELF-TALK: WHAT YOU THINK AND SAY ABOUT YOURSELF

Self-talk is what you say, either aloud or in your mind, in conversation with yourself. Zig Ziglar, author, salesman, and motivational speaker, defined the influence of self-talk when he said, "If you realized how powerful your thoughts are, you would never think a negative thought." This is a formidable statement and should give us pause. How we talk to and about ourselves matters big time.

Do you struggle with negative self-talk? Most of us do. I know I do! When I first started running marathons it wasn't unusual, in the middle of a race, for me to occasionally wonder, *"Don, what were you thinking when you signed up for this? This is tough!"* Thankfully, I've faced this nagging voice enough times to learn how to flip my internal script and turn my negative self-talk to positive self-talk. When self-doubt creeps in, my other, more encouraging voice kicks in and says, "*Don, trust your training. You can do this. Hang in there!*"

Your self-talk starts and ends with how you feel about yourself. Psychologist, educator, and author Dr. Martin Seligman at the University of Pennsylvania has said, "The way you talk to yourself can determine your emotions, how you feel about yourself on a minute-to-minute basis." Understand that your words and thoughts have power! In my training as a marathon coach, I've had participants who immediately tell me they can't run a marathon because they're overweight, out of shape, too old, uncoordinated, have bad knees, etc. Their negative talk has them defeated before they even start. You may have applied for a job, and in the back of your mind, determined that you'll never get it. Maybe you think

> Understand that your words and thoughts have power!

you're underqualified, overqualified, or that you don't have the right experience. In my own life, I avoided signing up for a triathlon because I convinced myself that I couldn't swim. The thought of swimming, particularly in open water, was terrifying. I was defeated, declaring that I didn't know how to swim. But I overcame this fear, signed up for a triathlon, and conquered the swim.

Is your self-talk raising you up or holding you back? Your thoughts or words can lead to success or failure, so be aware of your self-talk, and don't minimize its impact on your attitude. As a wise person once said, "Watch your thoughts, for they become words. Watch your words, for they become actions. Watch your actions, for they become habits. Watch your habits, for they become character. Watch your character, for it becomes your destiny." Few of us escape the impact of self-talk on our attitudes. Self-talk is often a reflection of how you feel about yourself. It is important to be aware of what you say or think about yourself. More often than not, what we believe becomes our reality.

HOW TO FLIP YOUR SCRIPT

So when the going gets tough—let's say you've recently lost your job—how do you turn those nagging, negative voices into more supportive self-talk?

1. Take a deep breath, hit the pause button, and remember your past successes. All is not lost. You're not a failure. Just because you lost your job doesn't mean you won't get another one.

2. Understand that you are resilient. You're stronger than you think. You *can* find another job. This is not the end of the world. The sun really will come up tomorrow. This, too, shall pass.

3. Don't be afraid to turn to the people around you for help. You can and should have a support system, and it's okay to ask for support now. Moreover, it's essential to ask for support.

CHANGE YOUR ATTITUDE, CHANGE YOUR LIFE

The bottom line: You can change your attitude and, in the process, change your life. My experience with cancer opened my eyes to the need to change the direction and priorities of my life. I was broken, realizing that I had the wrong priorities, motivations, and goals for my life. I had focused on work, making money, and the material items I could buy. I recall wanting a bigger house, a newer car, a pool in the backyard, and more. There is absolutely nothing wrong with these thoughts, but it became more a need than a want. I was guilty of turning a want into a need and missing the point entirely. And yes, I was trying

> The bottom line: You can change your attitude and, in the process, change your life.

to keep up with the Joneses. I recognized the factors that were impacting my life and decided to use my forward-looking, positive attitude to change the direction of my life. This wasn't easy, since I had to overcome my self-doubt that I might not be able to change. But I'd faced tougher obstacles in the past, and I knew I could rely on my attitude to get me through the moments of uncertainty.

Negative thinking can get in the way of making a beneficial change in your attitude. It can stop you from moving forward. Keep in mind that you can turn this thinking around. You can do almost anything, if you want it enough and are willing to strive for it. One of my favorite quotes from Napoleon Hill, author of personal success literature, offers reassurance that change is always possible: "What the mind can conceive and believe, the mind can achieve." There's no "right time." You can start changing your outlook at any time. Why not start right now? This very minute. Every day presents a window of opportunity for a change in your attitude.

My attitude evolved from the insight I gained in my early teens. Throughout my life, I've chosen a positive attitude over a negative attitude. My attitude served as my ally during my cancer fight. Basically, I was operating by instinct, but unquestionably the experience certainly tested me. My attitude was a game changer. You can experience the same type of success by changing your attitude to confront the next curveball that life throws at you.

It's important to recognize that your attitude will change, as you are confronted by and overcome life's adversity. We don't always comprehend or recognize a change while it's occurring, but it's happening nonetheless. It's worth spending some time assessing where your attitude is now in relationship to how you'd like it to be. Don't wait for a catastrophic event to force you to change. You have the power to change now.

> A change in your attitude can change the course and outcome of your life and the lives of those around you.

Events, circumstances, and experiences can change your attitude. A change in your attitude can change the course and outcome of your life and the lives of those around you. So, choose wisely. Choose to be positive! Choose to be successful! Don't be afraid to be awesome by changing a negative attitude to a positive attitude, and watch it change your life. Change your attitude and literally change the direction and success of your life!

CHAPTER 7

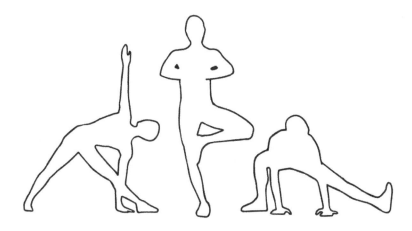

Finding Balance

"Balance is not something you find,
it's something you create."

—Jana Kingsford

I don't personally profess to have perfect balance. I've struggled with this concept for most of my adult life. It's painful to admit that. I certainly didn't know balance was important, much less that it was something I should work at. I assumed that if I worked hard, applied myself, took direction, and always asked for more responsibility, everything else in my life, professionally and personally, would fall into place. In my mind, there was nothing wrong with my workaholic tendencies. In fact, I didn't even recognize that I was a workaholic. It's how I'd been since I was twelve years old. I believed work was the driving force of a successful life and, therefore, it was my number-one priority.

In my early professional life, I generally worked seven days a week, every week, for the majority of the year. I didn't take vacations because who has time for vacations? I missed family events because of work commitments. I was absolutely convinced that if I was successful at work—meaning I made enough money to afford a home, car, and stuff—I would be loved and adored by all. Success at work, no matter the price, would translate into success in all other areas of my life.

Unfortunately, my understanding didn't change until I was faced with a life-threatening illness. I'm not saying I have all the answers now, but I have changed my perspective for the better. I realized that I needed to make an effort to bring balance and, ultimately, harmony into my life. I had to remind myself that I didn't live in a vacuum and there were other people in my life. Recognizing this was a monumental realization for me. I've since learned to nurture relationships and move away from a more self-centered way of living. In contrast to my young adulthood, a relationship-centered life now takes priority. Working seven days a week and always striving for more **does not** meet this criteria.

BALANCE DEFINED

Webster's dictionary defines "balance" as "a state of equilibrium or equipoise." In life, this definition of balance is hard to attain. Balance in real life doesn't mean dividing your time and energy equally among various areas of your life. This would not only be impractical but also impossible.

Trying to find balance might at times feel like spinning multiple plates in the air, as you might see in a circus act. It's difficult to find just the right number of plates to spin. At times, you're spinning too many plates and a few crash to the ground and shatter. At other times, you don't spin enough plates, and you can't keep up the momentum of those you do have spinning. The right balance of spinning plates is unique and different for everyone.

> Balance in real life doesn't mean dividing your time and energy equally among various areas of your life.

Everyone has different priorities, goals, and needs at various stages of life, and the time and energy you spend in each area of your life will inevitably shift over the years. Your priorities will shift multiple times over the course of your life. Relationships, marriage, children, work, retirement—these all denote different priorities. As a young adult, you may be focused on finishing your education and starting your career. Focusing most of your energy on your education at this point in your life doesn't make you out of balance—it's normal. There are certain periods of your life when one area may need most of your focus. In the weeks leading up to final exams, for example, studying will take priority, and in the months when you're training for a marathon, your training may require more time than evenings out with friends. However, this doesn't mean you should forget everything else around you—your family, friends, or health, for example.

Life balance is nebulous and difficult to consistently achieve. Some would argue that balance is impossible to accomplish. The point is, be aware of life balance and learn to be flexible with this concept. Try not to be too rigid in your efforts to maintain life balance. No single definition suits everyone, and each day has a slightly different feel in terms of what's right. For me, simply recognizing the concept of balance fundamentally changed the way I viewed the activities of my day. I realized that there is more to a day than the hours devoted to work. This gave me the insight (I know that sounds silly) to acknowledge the other valuable areas of my life. In other words, the importance of family and friends, recreation and fun.

Keep in mind that we are all really good at justifying what we are doing and how we are using our time. It's human nature to do so, to the point where we don't even consider the potential negative consequences of our actions. I was exceptionally adept at justifying my actions; for example, I had to work seven days a week because my job required my constant attention. One of the lessons I've learned in the past ten years—and *this* is important—is that we do, for the most part, exactly

> Keep in mind that we are all really good at justifying what we are doing and how we are using our time.

what we want to do, when we want to, and we don't take the time to think about or even explain our actions.

You may (now) be asking, when is your balancing act unbalanced?

1. You're up early in the morning; it's dark outside. You get ready for work and off you go. You work all day and come home when it's dark outside. You've been so busy, you really don't have a grasp of what happened at work, and you have even less knowledge of what's going on at home. You haven't seen your kids (awake) for days and probably missed their ball games, dance recitals, etc.

2. You spend your day taking your children from one activity to the other. You have no time to enjoy what they are doing because you're in the taxi business for your family. You may even forget who you are picking up and where they are supposed to go.

3. You don't have time to take care of daily living activities (paying bills, grocery shopping, seeing family and friends, etc.) because you are "too busy!"

4. You are so busy taking care of the household that you have no time to take care of you. You do nothing for you! You don't exercise, you don't eat right, you don't read, you don't relax, etc.

5. You spend hours on some form of electronic device (too many to mention) when you're home, ignoring family and friends, etc.

6. You ignore vacations and use the excuse that you "have to work."

7. Here's a big one: Your relationships start to fall apart because you are not dedicating enough time to nurturing them.

At the beginning of my career in the golf business, I truly believed that I needed to devote every single waking hour to my profession. My singular focus and dedication made sense, to a point. I was trying to establish myself in my field, advance my career, and eventually start my own business. But even when I no longer needed to make the same personal sacrifices to achieve my goals, I still found reasons to postpone investing in other parts of my life. I worked constantly, and sadly, I justified this approach to others and myself. I ignored virtually every other aspect of my life, including my family, friends, and health. I had few close friends, no hobbies, virtually no family vacations, and stranded marriages. "*I would have time tomorrow*," I rationalized, but tomorrow there was always a new reason to put my career first. It wasn't that I didn't have any fun; for me, work was fun. I just missed out on a fuller, more engaging, and vibrant life, and my relationships especially suffered. Work was my sole source of fulfillment, and I didn't question the way I was conducting my life until years later, after I had already experienced significant losses resulting from my choices. I talk a great deal about work because that was a driving force in my world. It is important to note that your source of self-satisfaction may not be work related. You may want to examine what it is for you.

> Your life balance is based on choices you make concerning how you use your time and energy.

So, what's the point? Your life balance is based on *choices* you make concerning how you use your time and energy. Until you closely examine how you invest your time and energy, you won't be able to match those choices to your true priorities and live a more balanced life. You probably don't have the same type of imbalance that I did. Everyone is different. You may even be unaware of how the choices you are making are significantly (and possibly negatively) affecting other areas of your life—particularly important relationships.

HOW YOUR BALANCING ACT IMPACTS OTHERS

If nothing else from this chapter sticks with you, remember this: Your approach to life balance has a significant impact on the people in your life. The Dalai Lama pretty much sums it up: "Just as ripples spread out when a single pebble is dropped into water, the actions of individuals can have far-reaching effects." If you choose, for example, to make your career the central focus of your life, as I did, the relationships in your life will be affected. It's unavoidable. You simply can't ignore an area (or areas) of your life and believe that these areas will thrive or that things will work themselves out. You can only miss so many of your kid's soccer games or piano recitals or cancel a certain number of dinner dates or weekend getaways with your significant other before it starts to take a toll. Relationships require time and nurturing to grow and remain meaningful. You don't live in a vacuum. Life balance is not possible if you focus solely on one area at the expense of others, even if you are wildly successful in that one area. Keep in mind, too, that even if you're not a so-called "workaholic," your life balance might be out of whack.

For caregivers, who spend much of their time nurturing others, life balance can also be difficult to obtain. This is because putting others before your own health or well-being indefinitely and completely can negatively affect your relationships. If you don't take care of yourself, eventually you won't be able to take care of anyone else either. Balance across all areas of your life is vital, in order to have successful relationships with others.

HOW BALANCED ARE YOU?

Life balance doesn't just happen for most people. You have to work at achieving it. You have to be committed to it. You also have to regularly reevaluate how you spend your time and energy as circumstances and your priorities change. In other words, ignoring life balance and hoping it will work itself out doesn't work.

On the other hand, don't overwhelm yourself with the mechanics of life balance. Not thinking about life balance is a problem but so is *overthinking* it. It's a process, not a destination. It doesn't mean having every moment of each day categorized and scheduled. Balance shouldn't be a frantic act of compulsively checking off the boxes in your life each day. Getting bogged down in the minutiae of achieving 100% life balance in every area of your life will only frustrate you. It's not possible. Just being aware of what life balance is and how to manage it, for you, is half the battle. Finding balance is about making a

> Getting bogged down in the minutiae of achieving 100% life balance in every area of your life will only frustrate you.

conscious effort to cultivate various areas of your life and not letting one area dominate the others for too long. Again, keep in mind that success in one area does not guarantee or equate to success in other areas. This was the mistake I made as a young adult, and it's taken years and several major challenges to correct it.

Since life balance is different for everyone, your decisions about what to prioritize and when will be unique to you. Achieving life balance involves personal investigation and self-discovery. Bottom line? Try to balance your time among the various areas of your life, but don't feel defeated if you don't meet this expectation. Achieving meaningful life balance will require regular self-assessments, commitment, and energy throughout your lifetime.

Four areas of life balance can serve as your starting point in your discovery process:

- Spiritual (God)
- Relationships (Family, Friends, and Acquaintances)
- Professional (Work)
- Recreational (Hobbies, Sports, and Fun)

This list is by no means all-inclusive. Your priorities might also include community leadership, volunteer work, and fitness—you fill in the blanks!

COMING BACK TO BALANCE

Life balance and, ultimately, harmony *can* exist in your life. Self-evaluation is a great starting point, and continued reevaluation is an ongoing and necessary process. Finding balance is a four-step process.

1.) **First and foremost,** *you must make life balance a priority.* In other words, you've got to recognize its importance and think about it as it relates to you. Once you've identified balance as something important to you and others around you, determine or identify what it means to you. Don't just talk about it; understand and commit to doing something about it.

2.) **Second, you need to** *identify* **what matters most to you by collecting information about how you currently spend your time.** You may think you have a good idea about how, when, and where you use your time and energy. My experience is that our perception isn't always in sync with how we *actually* spend our time and energy.

I went through a period of self-evaluation, and the results were surprising. I was especially surprised by how much time I wasted watching television or surfing the Internet. Productive moments were sandwiched in between a lot of wasted time. I believed I was very productive and always used my time wisely. Wow, was I wrong!

Start by completing the Life Balance Chart on the following page, which will help you see how you currently use your time and energy on a daily basis. Complete this process every day for one week so you have what I would call "a full cycle of activity." At the end of one week, you should have a good idea about your current priorities. When you see how you spend your days, you'll probably be rather surprised.

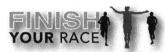 *Life Balance Chart*

	Sunday	Monday	Tuesday	Wednesday	Thursday	Friday	Saturday
6:00/7:00 am							
7:00/8:00 am							
8:00/9:00 am							
9:00/10:00 am							
10:00/11:00 am							
11:00/12:00 am/pm							
12:00/1:00 pm							
1:00/2:00 pm							
2:00/3:00 pm							
3:00/4:00 pm							
4:00/5:00 pm							
5:00/6:00 pm							
6:00/7:00 pm							
7:00/8:00 pm							
8:00/9:00 pm							
9:00/10:00 pm							
10:00/11:00 pm							
11:00/12:00 pm/am							

Life Balance Category Suggestions

- Work • Commuting - to & from work
- Carpooling - driving kids to & from activities
- Community volunteering • Church and/or
  associated activities
- Exercise/Fitness - working out in the gym, running,
  cycling, swimming, etc. • Hobbies - Reading, playing, etc.

- Meal prep & eating • Household chores laundry,
  dishes, cleaning, yard work, etc.
- Television/Computer - FaceBook, video games,
  Google searches, email, internet activities, etc.
- Paying bills

Go to **DonArmstrongLive.com** for a full size usable version of this chart

3.) **Third, you need to *evaluate* this information to determine whether you are spending your time in a way that is in harmony with what you value most.** So, did you complete the balance chart? Okay, looking over the information you collected for the past week, does anything jump out or shock you? Look for patterns and eye openers. For example, are you working constantly? Do you spend hours each day on Facebook? Are you spending zero time on physical fitness? Do you sleep four, five, six, or eight hours per night? Are you volunteering for everything at the expense of your family? What did you learn about yourself? Would you say the reality of your life (what you are actually doing) matches the priorities and values you believe you have in your head? If not, based on your Life Balance Chart what *are* you considering as a priorities? The first time I completed the chart my priorities contradicted the beliefs in my head. I was shocked at where I was devoting my time.

Even if you aren't happy with what you found in this life balance evaluation, take heart. You are drawing closer to a better understanding of life balance, simply by paying attention to how you spend your time. Analyzing how you spend your time is essential for a number of reasons. First, it will help you identify the areas of your life you consider important, versus those that you believe are important. Second, the process will clearly show the time and energy you currently dedicate to each of these areas and will subsequently help you determine where balance is lacking. Third, it will provide you with insight about possible adjustments you can make.

4.) **Finally, if you find that your life is out of balance, you can find ways to *improve* your connection with life balance.** There is no one-size-fits-all, plug-and-play approach to achieving life balance that works for everyone. However, if you feel pulled too far in one direction, you may be out of balance. What you are looking for is a comfortable state of equilibrium, not perfect harmony all the time. Do you have a better idea now of which aspects of your life aren't being attended to and nurtured? I hope so! This process was invaluable to me.

The easiest way to move toward a more balanced life is to first and foremost eliminate activities that zap your time and energy yet don't contribute to your quality of life, such as mindless Internet, email, and television viewing, among other things. Identify the areas that drain your time and eliminate them from your life, little by little or all at once. Just like you have the power to choose your attitude, you have the power to choose how you spend your time. This was huge for me, as I worked to improve balance in my life.

Be mindful that in your quest to find balance, it's important to check in with yourself. In other words, are you doing something for yourself every day? This is important for all of us. If not, make an appointment with yourself! You make an appointment for everything else in your life that's important. It's common, though, for us to forget ourselves in the scheduling process. So, we have to schedule time for ourselves. In the process of writing this book, I had to schedule time to write. Sounds strange, I know, but when I didn't, it wasn't unusual for me to run out of time in my day. Set aside time every day for an activity you enjoy: running, reading, meditating, or listening to music.

Are you scheduling time with your significant other? Do you schedule a date night? One of the things I've always admired about my brother is his 35-year commitment to Friday night date night with his wife. That's balance at work in a relationship. Do you set aside time to spend with your kids? Yes, put it on your schedule. Although this sounds as if you have to schedule time with your children out of obligation, putting it on the calendar simply reminds you to dedicate time with them rather than doing something else.

Once you've scheduled time for you, schedule time for your family, your friends, your health, and your work. Understand that your work hours are generally set so these hours will go on your chart first. Realize that work is not the only activity of your day. And overachievers, listen up: You must learn to say "No!" You can't volunteer for everything. And you can't do everything for everyone.

After you make adjustments in the time and energy you are devoting to specific areas of your life balance, track your progress in the areas you identified. In other words, determine your success in rebalancing your life by simply charting another week. This will make tracking your progress easy. Compare the new week's chart to your original chart. Progress will jump out at you and will be easy to see and quantify. To double check your findings, have a trusted family member or friend rate you on the areas that are important to you. This should be an open, two-way conversation. Compare the results of this conversation. Are they similar? Ask yourself what areas still need improvement in order to better balance your time and energy.

Life is crazy for all of us. Balance, if we are even aware of the concept, is a challenge we all face to one degree or another. There are days when we feel in perfect balance and days we feel totally out of balance. We are constantly adjusting our schedules to meet the demands of our lives, work, family, etc. Part of living a balanced life also means trying to live in

> There are days when we feel in perfect balance and days we feel totally out of balance.

balance and make room for unforeseen circumstances, uncertainty, and adversity, without those hardships overtaking your life and overwhelming you.

A FINAL WORD ON BALANCE

What did I learn about my own life balance in my journey? Simply put, I learned that work is not the be-all and end-all. This was an extremely painful, unexpected revelation, which was difficult for me to grasp until relationships I thought were solid faltered. Success at work by no means translated into success in the other areas of my life. In fact, the other areas of my life were often a disaster.

I learned that to be a fulfilled, happy, and successful individual, I needed to think about balance and invest in all segments of my life. It's not about giving each area equal time down to the minute, but it is about engaging and committing to giving every relevant priority a prominent place in my life. I couldn't let one area dominate my life anymore. That meant that I needed to work hard, apply myself, take direction, and always ask for more to be successful in *all* areas of my life, not just in my professional sphere.

I now understand that when I leave this earth, no one will comment on how much money I made, where I lived, what I drove, or how I vacationed. Instead, I will be remembered for how much of a difference I made in other people's lives. In other words, I will be remembered for the relationships in my life. So put your energy where it matters most. Work on life balance for yourself, but also work on it for the important people with whom you share your life. They will thank you for it.

> Work on life balance for yourself, but also work on it for the important people with whom you share your life.

CHAPTER 8

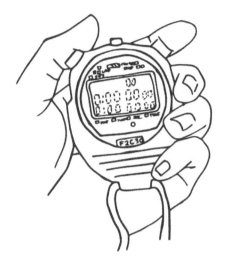

Understanding Expectations— Yours and Others

"A wonderful gift may not be wrapped as you expect."

—Jonathan Lockwood Huie

Prior to my cancer diagnosis, I really didn't give much serious consideration to expectations. But like you, I had them. I expected, for example, to graduate from high school and go to college. I had an expectation for my college experience, and of course, I expected to graduate and get a job. I had an expectation about what work would be like, what my career would be, and how successful I'd become. I also had an expectation about marriage and what it would look like.

Unfortunately, I didn't always share my expectations with anyone. Yet, I expected everyone in my world to know, sense, or understand what I was thinking. Sounds like a simple expectation, doesn't it? I certainly didn't think that others would have their own expectations to complicate mine. I also didn't think their expectations would be different from mine. Of course, I am kidding, however, I never gave much consideration to expectations in my life. This turned out to be a huge disconnect between me and just about everyone in my life. Nope, I had to learn the hard way that everyone has expectations and they do, in fact, matter.

Even if we don't consciously recognize them, we have expectations for everyone, including ourselves, and for every event in our lives. Your expectations may be realistic or unrealistic; however, they are your own, and they have a profound impact on how you view and react to the world and others in your life. Expectations can be simple, such as expecting the lights to come on when you flip the light switch, expecting your car to start when you turn the key, or expecting a paycheck at the end of a pay period. We expect these things to happen in a certain way and only really think about them when they don't.

Generally speaking, your expectations are based on your beliefs. The main problem with this is, like an iceberg, 90% of your beliefs and expectations are hidden from your awareness, while you tend to regard the remaining 10%—the expectations you are aware of—as valid and realistic. Whether they're simple or complicated, your expectations usually only step into the limelight when you're happily surprised or sorely disappointed with an outcome. Quite often, the expectations we put on ourselves can be unrealistic. In addition, we have a tendency to be our own toughest critic. I know I was!

Whether it was at work or at home, my limited understanding and acknowledgement of expectations—both my own and others'—led me to believe that I was on the right path. I *had* to be doing the right thing, the best thing, for my family and myself, based on my expectations. In certain areas of my life, particularly in my intimate relationships, my expectations were seldom met. Remember, I thought I was on the right path, so I couldn't be wrong. And when these relationships would go off track, I would be reminded of Albert

> Your expectations usually only step into the limelight when you're happily surprised or sorely disappointed with an outcome.

Einstein's definition of insanity: doing the same thing over and over again and expecting different results. I kept trying to fix the problem (which of course couldn't be me; Ha!) by moving to a new relationship and trying again. I've joked that I haven't been good at picking partners, but the fact is, I had unrealistic and poorly communicated expectations in my relationships. So while I shouldn't have expected different results, I did.

As a young man, I had sincere thoughts, hopes, and dreams that were meaningful to me. I'm not sure why, but I assumed that everyone around me could read my mind or was somehow connected to what I was thinking, where I was going, and what I wanted. Maybe I believed everyone agreed with me or that they wanted the same things I did. Somehow, someway, I got by for a while without talking through my thoughts and ideas with those closest to me. Open, honest communication could have saved me from a lot of disappointment and heartache.

It was important for me to include a chapter on expectations because my lack of understanding them led me astray for most of my life, and I don't want the same thing to happen to you. I'm certain I can't be the only person who has endured unrealized or misplaced expectations. I learned early in life to look for the positive in almost every circumstance, and I generally expected everything would always be okay. I certainly didn't expect to wake up with leukemia in 2005, any more than I expected to wake up jobless or in a relationship that was ending. Like me, you also have expectations about how you should be, how other people should be, and how your life should be.

Fortunately, my diagnosis with leukemia prompted me to examine almost every area of my life, and I had the chance to give my expectations a long, hard look. After a good deal of pain and loss, I had come to truly believe Shakespeare when he said, "Expectation is the root of all heartache." While failing to manage expectations can bring heartache and stress, I was equally confident that communicating and realizing expectations could bring great joy and blessings. No doubt, I had a lot to learn—and a lot of work to do.

WHERE DO YOUR EXPECTATIONS COME FROM?

Expectations aren't developed in a vacuum. Once again, they are most often based on past experiences. In other words, an expectation is essentially a preconceived outlook for how our circumstances should turn out and what we think will bring us either success or failure, happiness or disappointment. They shape not only how we interpret outcomes but also the emotions we have around outcomes and the conclusions we draw from them about what to expect in the future.

Expectations are derived from your life experiences from the day you are born. As a result, expectations have roots in your childhood and early adult experiences. Your parents, relatives, and close family friends have a significant impact on early expectations. Not only are your expectations affected by your upbringing, they are also affected by your education, career training, and your understanding of laws and social norms. Expectations represent your beliefs, wants, and desires, and they live mostly in your subconscious. Expectations will often change and evolve over time, as you grow and mature in response to life's circumstances.

> Expectations are derived from your life experiences from the day you are born.

Here's one example of how past experience led to future expectations. My early work experience at Winterwood Golf Club exposed me to a group of individuals who I considered family. The Huff and Breaux families taught me, at a very young age, the value of working hard and applying myself. They instilled in me a strong work ethic and also created an expectation in me that hard work results in success. This early foundation helped me to understand a path to succeed in my career. It also showed me the value and benefit of a single-minded focus in achieving career goals and ultimately success.

My Winterwood family also imparted to me the power of positive thinking. I learned by watching their example. They didn't just tell me, they also showed me what positive thinking could do, which was far more effective. They didn't just talk about the concept; they lived it every day. They always had a smile on their faces and a kind or encouraging word for everyone, if the situation called for it. I admired them and wanted to emulate them. Joe LePire, the assistant golf professional at Winterwood, had a significant influence on developing my positive attitude and encouraged me to read self-help books. In fact, the first books I read were Norman Vincent Peale's *The Power of Positive Thinking* and Napoleon Hill and W. Clement Stone's *Success Through a Positive Mental Attitude*. Experiencing this type of thinking and seeing it firsthand made a significant impact on me at a young age. These early experiences resulted in an expectation that all things were possible if you worked hard and believed in yourself.

> Expectations play an important role in how we encounter life and can have a profound impact on our career, relationships, health, and mental well-being.

I share this example because it illustrates how expectations can be a driving factor in your happiness, joy, and success. Expectations play an important role in how we encounter life and can have a profound impact on our career, relationships, health, and mental well-being. Expectations can empower us, but they can also be disempowering or contribute to an out-of-kilter life balance. And, unfortunately, when your expectations are unfulfilled, it can sometimes lead to feelings of anger, frustration, and even depression.

THE POWER OF YOUR PAST

Expectations are tricky to negotiate because your past is a powerful thing. At this point in your journey, you've developed your own unique preconceptions about outcomes, based on your specific life experiences. Expectations are truly in the eye of the beholder. Your expectations don't always match the expectations of others, which can make relationships difficult. Differences in expectations can lead to disappointments in different areas of your life, including home, work, and friendships. When your expectations are not met, your negative feelings can feel much stronger than the good feelings we get when our expectations are exceeded. When circumstances don't meet your expectations, your brain doesn't just grumble, it sends out a message of possible DANGER and FEAR.

It is important to be aware of the expectations you hold, both for yourself and others. You certainly can't insist that others accept your expectations without a conversation and mutual agreement. You also can't assume that they understand what your expectations are without a discussion. No one is a mind reader (recall my own previously mentioned disappointing conclusion). It's essential to recognize that people in our lives may have expectations for us they haven't communicated, either. Together, you can and should acknowledge and discuss differences in expectations.

HOW EXPECTATIONS AND
REALITY ALIGN—OR DON'T

Remember the quote at the beginning of the chapter? "A wonderful gift may not be wrapped as you expect." As soon as we see a package, we develop an expectation of what's inside. We shake the package to listen for a familiar sound, we use size to guess what's inside, and we may even sniff or feel around the package. We use all of our senses to determine what's inside. But we don't always get what we hoped for, wanted, or expected.

I experienced a profound sense of pain and disappointment around the tenth month of my battle with cancer. I had been through the challenges of treatment, and recovery was in sight. My wife had been by my side literally every step of the way, from the minute of my diagnosis. She was there for every doctor's appointment, every bone marrow aspiration and biopsy, and every round of chemo. She took notes from conversations with doctors, nurses, and social workers. She set her work schedule around my treatment and rearranged her life to spend every single night with me in the hospital. She slept sixty plus nights on a pullout chair bed close to my bed. She was always there and always doing everything possible to make sure I was okay. She was, in a word, *amazing.*

She even took care of many uncomfortable situations. For example, I wasn't thrilled with my first oncologist. His bedside manner and general attitude, I felt, left something to be desired. During the morning of my second day at Harris Hospital, my doctor was on vacation, so a different doctor came in to visit with me. I liked his demeanor and how he devoted time to talk with me, asking if I had any questions. My wife immediately sensed the change in my attitude with this doctor and asked, "You like him, don't you?" I said, "Yes!" Out the door she went. Five minutes later, she reappeared with a smile on her face: "You have a new doctor!" Without me having to say a word, she knew I was thrilled!

I never expected that my wife would decide to end our relationship after everything we'd gone through, especially now when I was finally on the real road to recovery. Nothing in the previous ten months could have prepared me for this reality. She had been my rock, and yet our experiences had not been the same. She was grateful that I was doing well, but she was worn out and spent. It was time for her to move on, and there was nothing I could do about it. This was certainly an unmet expectation for me. In many ways, this was more difficult to deal with than the cancer itself.

HOW TO KEEP YOUR EXPECTATIONS IN CHECK

Every time I run a marathon, I expect to finish within a certain time frame. My goal is based on how much effort or time I put into training, which, if any, injuries I may have sustained, and how I feel on race day. I don't always meet my expectations. Sometimes the weather, how I'm feeling, or difficult course conditions force me to let go of my expectations. When I cross the finish line and see my time, I try to understand that reality doesn't always square up with what I think should happen, and that not every component of my daily life is within my control.

Keeping your expectations in check can save you a lot of frustration. Being realistic about expectations doesn't mean you expect bad outcomes. Cynically, I've heard people say that you should expect less so as not to be disappointed. But in my experience, I believe that you should always expect the best in all circumstances. As Norman Vincent Peale wrote, "Shoot for the moon. Even if you miss, you'll land among the stars."

Expectations may not always align with reality, but they do affect your reality. When I received my cancer diagnosis, I didn't really know what to expect. But I knew I had a choice, and I chose positivity. Really, what else could I choose? I expected to survive, so I acted like I would survive. I kept my expectations positive and never allowed myself to consider the negative consequences of my diagnosis. Although this was certainly easier said than done, in the long run, this approach made all the difference for me. There are no guarantees in life, remember? Expect the unexpected, and expect that hardship will find you sometime. No one is immune to this possibility. But again, no matter how dire your circumstances might feel, you always have a choice. So, embrace your expectations wisely with a complete understanding of what they mean to you and others.

> Expectations may not always align with reality, but they do affect your reality.

During my first hospital stay, I expected to maintain a normal life, at least as much as I could while isolated on the seventh floor of Harris Hospital. I couldn't even get on the elevator, go downstairs, and take a walk outside, as there was too much of a risk for infection. Believe me, I tried, but the nurses always stopped me. But even with that restriction, I was determined to make the experience as routine as possible.

In the early days of my leukemia, I asked a lot of questions, like how long I could expect to be in the hospital. I heard one week from my doctor—or maybe that's what I wanted to hear. My nurse, however, quickly corrected my misunderstanding and prepared me to expect a stay of three to four weeks. She told me that acute leukemia patients typically have long hospital stays due to a side effect of treatment, an increased risk of infection. After getting over the shock, I thought, *"How can I make this month as normal as possible?"* So I asked my nurse what a typical day was like and what I could expect. When is breakfast? When does the doctor come by my room? What about lunch? And dinner? It seemed like a lot revolved around when the next meal was scheduled to arrive. There was always an expectation of what the meal would be and, more importantly, whether I would have the stomach to handle it. So yes, mealtime was a big deal.

I *expected* to maintain a regular routine while in the hospital, so I got up early every morning, shaved, and showered before breakfast exactly like I would have in my life before my treatment. I *expected* to see my doctor when I was dressed and ready for the day, just like I would have before my first meeting of the business day. I determined on day one that I would not wear a hospital gown. Several nurse techs insisted that I wear a gown, but I declined. My daily uniform was a pair of shorts and a golf shirt. My doctor would usually visit with me around seven. This was the first big moment of each day: something to be prepared for and look forward to each day. After this visit, I would get out of my hospital bed and usually sit in a chair next to the window. I had a panoramic view of Fort Worth from my seventh floor window. In my life pre-treatment life, I rarely watched TV during the day so that option was out of the question. Instead I would read a book (a new hobby for me) or visit with friends and family.

Despite my efforts to make life in the hospital normal, my expectations of each day didn't always match up with how my day turned out. Treatment sometimes made me groggy or nauseous, and some days I didn't feel so good. I slowly learned to adapt. After all, had my expectations for this experience been written in stone, I would have been disappointed on a daily basis. I just had to take it moment by moment. If life couldn't be "normal" one day, maybe it would be the next. I always *expected* the best.

EXPRESS YOURSELF

Actively managing expectations is critical to creating better outcomes, and mastering this strategy will ultimately lead to a more fulfilling life. Doing this involves eliminating the gap between what you expect and what actually happens. Your expectations must be both realistic and clearly communicated to be managed. How we manage expectations is critical to how we view our experiences, pursue our goals, and define our success. As automatic or reflexive as they can sometimes feel, it's important to understand your expectations and from where they originate. This awareness will allow you to decide if they are worth keeping or if it's time to change them. Unless you are aware of your expectations, you can't change them, and you certainly can't communicate them to yourself or others.

> If life couldn't be "normal" one day, maybe it would be the next. I always expected the best.

Once you are aware of your own expectations, shift your attention to understanding others' expectations. Keep in mind, this isn't possible without communication. Communicate early and often. Expectations are a two-way street, and expectations that are seldom discussed often will lead to disappointment. Discuss the reasons for both your expectations and others'. Take a moment to assess whether your expectations are *realistic, reasonable, and clear.* This is not the time to disguise your true feelings. You don't have to agree on all expectations, but you need to communicate your expectations so the other person understands what you are thinking and why. This forms the foundation for empathy and is especially important should a major crisis or hardship arise. At the heart of managing our expectations is the need to respect each other's differences and to endeavor to see situations from someone else's point of view.

Communicating expectations involves listening. I am talking about active, not passive, listening. You have got to listen with both ears, giving your undivided attention to the other person, rather than merely thinking about your response while the other person talks. Let them know you're listening by reflecting back what they've told you. You don't have to agree with everything they say, but I would urge you to keep an open mind and reserve judgment. Don't assume that you know someone else's expectations before you sit down to talk through them together. I was a master at this, and you can see where it got me. Don't plan on your expectations always matching up, either. Keep in mind that you can only control your own expectations. It's also important to talk about *mutual* expectations, including needs, wants, desires, and planned outcomes.

If you sense that someone's expectations are not realistic, achievable, or plausible, sharing your concerns is okay and sometimes very necessary. Nothing can harm a relationship or frustrate someone you care for as quickly as unreasonable expectations. Keep talking, keep listening to each other, and keep working toward a realistic scenario. You must work at this process; it won't happen on its own. And please, take it from someone who's made a few mistakes: Managing expectations through consistent and clear communication isn't easy. Yet, it is absolutely necessary.

KEYS TO ADJUSTING YOUR EXPECTATIONS

Take some time to sit down and think about your expectations for various aspects of your life including college, work, marriage, family, parenthood, friendships, health, recreation, fitness, hobbies, and retirement. Once you've thought about these expectations, write down what you discover about yourself in as much detail as possible. Use the Expectations Chart on the following page to record your findings.

FINISH YOUR RACE   *Expectation Chart*

	Expectation(s)	Your Expectation	Origin of Expectation	Other's Expectation	Differences	Resolution/ Understanding
College						
Work						
Marriage						
Family						
Parenthood						
Friendships						
Health						
Recreation/Fitness						
Hobbies/Fun						
Retirement						

Go to **DonArmstrongLive.com** for a full size usable version of this chart

Write down your expectations. For example, regarding my work, I expected to get a job out of college as an assistant golf course superintendent, excel at the job, get promoted to a golf course superintendent position, make more money over time, and be considered a leader in my industry.

Consider the origin of your expectations. Can you recall specifically what event or events led to your expectation? For example, my Dad worked hard as an Air Force officer and pilot. He excelled at his work, was promoted, and moved up in rank. This made an impression on me and set the expectation that if you work hard and excel at your job you will advance in your career.

The next step is important and an absolute must: Compare your expectations with the expectations of the important people in your life. In other words, compare your expectations for a specific life area (work, marriage, family, etc.) with the expectations of an important person in your life, such as your spouse. How are they the same, and how do they differ? Discuss the similarities and differences to have a better understanding of that person and your relationship with each other.

It's okay to question your expectations to add clarity and certainty. It's also okay to consider and ensure that your expectations are genuine, achievable, and realistic. Do they reflect what you truly believe? Ask someone you trust to confirm that your expectations are genuine, achievable, and realistic. Do they sync with the expectations of the people in your life? If you have areas of frustration and disappointment in your life, write these down. Make sure you communicate and discuss these expectations with those who are affected by them. These feelings could very well be the result of unmet or unrealistic expectations.

Review your expectations periodically to make sure they still hold true for you. Expectations will more than likely change and evolve over time, so don't be afraid to adjust your expectations often and when appropriate. When a conflict results from unfilled expectations, stop and think before reacting. Be realistic when expectations—either your own or someone else's—are not met. Understand that expectations are at times influenced by circumstances that are out of your control, and try to adjust accordingly.

Don't set your expectations so high as to be out of reach, but don't set them too low, either, just to play it safe. If we make expectations too high, we set ourselves up for disappointment. If we make expectations too low, we risk living with an attitude of futility. I believe strongly in under promising and over delivering, and always going the extra mile to exceed someone else's expectations, if you can. With your expectations thoughtfully managed, you'll be rewarded with rich relationships and a deep sense of satisfaction.

If expectations of others are not genuine, realistic, and achievable, politely pushing back is okay and sometimes necessary. Nothing can demotivate you as quickly as unreasonable expectations with no chance to succeed. Keep working until you reach an equilibrium that works for all parties involved.

At the end of the day, your ability to manage expectations is going to be based on how well you communicate. If you leave details up to chance, chances are you will be disappointed. On the other hand, if you take the time to listen, proactively communicate in an open manner, and address concerns head on, you will keep expectations in check and be in a good position to grow satisfying relationships over time.

> At the end of the day, your ability to manage expectations is going to be based on how well you communicate.

There is no template for managing expectations, other than the fact that you should be aware of your own expectations and how they meet or compare to the expectations of others. You must work at this process, as it won't happen on its own. Managing expectations, through consistent communication, will lead to better outcomes with fewer disappointments. Finally, it seems best to have low expectations for things that are out of your control and realistic expectations for things you can control.

CHAPTER 9

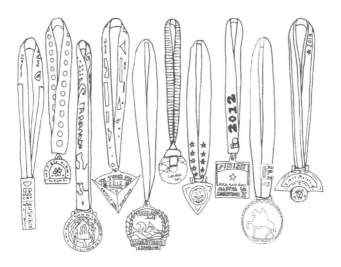

Combining Purpose
with Passion

*"Purpose is the reason you journey. Passion
is the fire that lights your way."*

—Unknown

Why do you get up in the morning? Sure, you want to get to your job, class, or other responsibilities. But there may be something bigger that energizes you. Your all-caps, boldface **WHY**! What makes you feel fulfilled, deeply satisfied, and impresses on you that you're contributing to something greater than yourself? Maybe you already know what your *Why* is, or maybe, like I had, you've lost your sense of connection to it. Maybe you haven't yet started to discover it. Your *Why* is your purpose and it's yours alone. Only you can determine it.

Napoleon Hill defines purpose as "the starting point of all achievement, and its lack is the stumbling block for ninety-eight out of every hundred people simply because they never really define their goals and start toward them." And it's true. Purpose is powerful! It will energize your thinking morning, noon, and night. It's what will give you hope for your future and allow you to see the big picture of your life. Purpose will inspire you and motivate you to keep going when you reach a stumbling block. Purpose will keep you on target and help you overcome obstacles, real and imagined, ultimately enabling you to see the infinite potential in your world. Purpose guides your actions and gives clear direction to your life. Purpose is the driving force in your life that will lead your every step forward.

Purpose wakes you every morning ready to tackle the day. When you tap into your sense of purpose, you won't even think about hitting the snooze button on your alarm clock. At the end of a long, exhausting day, purpose keeps you going even if you have no more to give. It might even keep you up late at night—in the best way. As I wrote this book, I experienced a strong sense of purpose. Many nights, I was so absorbed in this project that I completely lost track of time.

Purpose is that powerful!

GETTING TO MY WHY

As I mentioned in a previous chapter, my battle against leukemia led me—quite unexpectedly—to reflect on the purpose of my life. In the long days I spent at the hospital and in the weeks I spent recovering from treatment and GVHD, I was surprised to hear a persistent voice in my mind, one I hadn't heard since I was a young adult. *"Why am I here? Where am I going? What's important to me? How am I making a difference?"* Maybe you know this voice. It lives inside all of us, but some of us do a great job of confining it in some dusty, cobweb-filled corner of our mind. I certainly had.

It was difficult for me to realize that I simply didn't have answers to some of these questions. Those answers I did have felt hollow. Although I had been successful in my life professionally,

> Purpose guides your actions and gives clear direction to your life.

the where, what, why, and how of my world felt very distant from me. Even though I had accomplished a great deal and was considered successful, I didn't feel fulfilled. I felt like something huge was missing from my life. Turns out my priorities, motivations, and goals weren't truly adding value to anyone's life, including mine.

My leukemia diagnosis made me second-guess or rethink almost every aspect of my life. During this period of reflection (remember all those miles I was running and the thinking I accomplished), I spent a great deal of time asking myself questions about my life's purpose. Lots of questions! I wanted to know what made me tick and why. I wanted to know if my motivations were authentic to me.

Facing a life-threatening illness had brought me to a major cross-road I never thought I'd come to in my life. Answering some important questions—maybe the *most* important questions—required me to dig deep, to be honest and open with myself, to get up close and personal with aspects of myself that I barely recognized. It felt like meeting a new person—awkward and a little uncomfortable. But once I got to know this other side of me a bit better, I realized without a doubt that I needed to change the direction of my life. I needed to discover my purpose, my burning reason, my *Why,* and power it with the energy and determination of a passion that was unstoppable.

So, I began the quest to find my purpose and the force of passion for my life. But I had no idea where to begin. I wasn't even sure I understood the meaning of purpose and passion. I questioned whether they were the same. I knew these two words are often used interchangeably and that other words like "intent" and "vision" were often thrown in the discussion—which frankly confused me. It was important to understand the meaning of these words, particularly if I was going to define them for me. I don't profess to be an expert on these two words, however, I have arrived at a definition that makes sense to me and hopefully to you.

FINDING YOUR PURPOSE

One's sense of purpose is not always easy to discover. There's a lot in your life competing for that top-of-mind prime real estate, and it's easy for purpose to get crowded out and retreat to those dark, cobwebby corners. For some people, it's not a priority, and for others, the motions of life day after day become so habitual they never feel the need to dig deeper. Like I did prior to my cancer diagnosis, some people feel their status quo is as good as it's going to get. But as with my experience, reaching one of life's major crossroad can provide you with a place to pause and reflect. The beauty of purpose, however, just like a positive attitude,

> The beauty of purpose, however, just like a positive attitude, is that it's always accessible to you if you choose to make space for it in your life.

is that it's always accessible to you if you choose to make space for it in your life. Unlike me, you don't have to spend ten months fighting cancer to find it.

Make no mistake: Finding your purpose will require you to dig deep. Purpose is not always easy to determine in your life. In fact, it may be difficult to find and may take time to identify. You may find yourself in uncharted waters, as you overcome some longstanding preconceptions about yourself in life—ideas you might have held onto for a long time. This will require you to ask and answer a lot of introspective questions. You will need to be honest with yourself. No matter what, keep looking. Your purpose is within you. It may be rusty from years of neglect, but it's there. Finding it might not be easy, but it will be worth it.

DIGGING DEEP

Getting to my own *Why* took a while. I started in July 2006, after my wife unexpectedly left me. This crushed me, and in many ways was as difficult as the leukemia treatment. Running became my therapy soon after my wife decided to leave. I actually thought through most of my big questions while I was running—that's when my thinking is clearest. It wasn't until June 2007, however, that my purpose started to become clear to me. That was when I went to my first Team in Training event, the San Diego Rock 'n' Roll Marathon. I was encouraged and inspired by all the people running together as one team to find a cure for blood cancer. Because of the selfless commitment I witnessed, I knew then that I had to do whatever I could to make a difference in other people's lives, since I was given back mine.

So now it's your turn to do some soul searching and find your race. Ready? Let's get started by thinking through the following questions and exploring your authentic, true self. Don't skip over any of these questions without writing down an answer. I really would like you to participate in this process. I don't want to drag you along with me. I really want this writing exercise to set you up for your success!

For some of you, this is going to be fun and exciting. For others, this may make you feel anxious or maybe even frustrated. Either way, it's okay! This is a moment of self-discovery that is 100% for you! Release any fear you may have about this process and keep an open mind.

Grab a journal, find a quiet space, and let your mind settle. You might take five or ten minutes to just sit in silence, breathe deeply, or meditate. The following exercise may take some time, and if you need to let these questions simmer and come back to them later, that's okay.

Here we go:

1. Is there something you've always dreamed of doing in your life? Is there a dream from your past (locked in your heart and head) that you've all but forgotten? Something you want to do within your lifetime? Something you are not currently doing? Focus on the dream!

2. What did you love doing as a child? Playing outside? Spending time with playmates? Reading books? Drawing? Games?

3. If you had all the money you needed, what would you do to contribute to the world? What would you do for absolutely no pay?

4. What do you absolutely love to do? What gives you joy and excitement? What would you happily devote hours doing if you had all the time in the world?

5. What are you good at without even trying? What are your talents and gifts? What makes you feel terrific about yourself?

6. What do you enjoy talking about with friends, family, and colleagues? What do you enjoy reading, researching, or studying? What do you Google?

7. When was the last time you felt excited? Exhilarated? What was the source of this feeling? Were you excited because of what you were doing?

8. What do you hope to do with your life? What is the one accomplishment you would like to achieve before the end of your life? What would you regret not doing, being, or having in your life?

9. What "cause" motivates you to volunteer? What would you like to do to improve your corner of the world? Will your "cause" make a difference in your life or, more importantly, someone else's life? Both?

10. What would your friends and family say you're good at doing? What would they say are your dreams and hopes? Is there something others ask you to help them with on a frequent basis? Take the time to ask your friends for feedback.

Still with me? Great! Your answers to the above questions are just the beginning of knowing and understanding yourself and your race in life. Hopefully, the answers to these questions will bring you closer to discovering your purpose. If nothing else, I hope this exercise started to get some ideas flowing, but if your purpose didn't come to you instantly, don't worry. Give it time, and keep revisiting these questions. Here's the powerful part about taking the time to discover (or rediscover) your purpose: When your purpose comes to you, and I believe it

> When your purpose comes to you, and I believe it will, you will feel truly unstoppable.

will, you will feel truly unstoppable. You'll feel excited about your life and ready to take on the world. Your life will have true meaning, and you will know the meaning of fulfillment through *your* purpose!

WHAT IS PASSION?

Passion is an intense emotion! In fact, it may be your most important asset. I would call it your secret sauce, like McDonald's has for the Big Mac. Passion is an energy force and an energy source. Passion supports your purpose. Purpose is the marriage of passion and action. It's the fuel that moves you forward every single day. It can act as your key to success and help get you through difficult times. A true and real passion (this is an action word) is natural and tireless. You can't fake real passion. It's something you feel and know. Consequently, others feel your passion. You either have it for something or you don't. We all know people who try to muster passion for something, but they just don't really feel it. They try to convince themselves, and maybe you, of their passion. This may last for a while, but eventually their words and actions fall flat. If your passion for something is real, instinct truly takes over. Passion is what allows you to stay focused, energized, and engaged with your sense of purpose.

PURPOSE CAN POWER YOUR LIFE

I understand if you are thinking, "*Wow, I'd love to leave my job to follow my purpose, but get real. I have bills to pay and a boss to answer to at work.*" You might feel trapped, or maybe you've settled so deeply into a comfort zone that it's hard to imagine changing your status quo to serve your purpose. Fear, doubt, and distractions will intensify these feelings and hold you back. If you're in the midst of major uncertainty, you might feel like your future is already pre-determined and it can't be changed. I understand, as I've had that exact mindset. Yet, isn't this your self-talk (thinking) holding you back with fear and doubt? This thinking can be changed, and you can make this happen with a profound purpose that moves you forward every day.

It's all too common to feel stuck in survival mode. It might even, in some way, feel comfortable, easy, or routine. Henry David Thoreau, author and philosopher, wrote, "Most men lead lives of quiet desperation and go to the grave with the song still in them." I believe that many individuals have this sense of longing to do more or be more in their life. I appreciate this and realize it is a real feeling. Some of you might just be discovering your sense of purpose. Hopefully, the questions above stirred something in you! You know that despite your day-to-day responsibilities, there is a greater reason for your life. But you might worry about what others would say, or maybe there's a voice in your head telling you that even if you gave it a try, you'd fail. You might feel like you lack the time, money, or financial security to chase down your purpose. Now this is important and hard: Ask yourself if you're playing it safe? Does the thought of doing what you *really* want scare you a little bit? Is your true purpose burning inside you, maybe way down deep, but you don't know what to do with it?

Here's what you should understand: Living with purpose doesn't mean doing something as drastic as quitting your job, moving to a new place, or becoming someone completely different. It does mean recognizing what's keeping you from living with purpose and doing something with conscious action, commitment, and dedication to overcome this feeling or thought. You'll probably need to step out of your comfort zone to do this, but you don't have to completely reinvent yourself.

You'll probably have some starts and stops, as you search for your purpose. You may find that what you thought was your purpose turns out to be nothing but a dead end. That's okay! Finishing your race is about understanding that it's never too late to change your life. Don't quit. Keep searching because once you tap into your purpose, the results will change your life forever. When you understand your life's purpose, you will be exuberantly passionate about it. You'll want to shout it from the rooftops, and you'll feel great that you're making a difference for yourself and others.

> Living with purpose doesn't mean doing something as drastic as quitting your job, moving to a new place, or becoming someone completely different.

PURPOSE SHOULD GUIDE YOUR LIFE!

Many of you may feel trapped in a comfort zone that won't allow you to follow your purpose. Your obligations keep you in a stagnant place, just because it's uncomfortable to change. Fears, self-doubt, and distractions in your life will intensify your trapped feeling and hold you back. As a result, you may feel your future is uncertain or already set in stone.

Are you so busy in your daily life that you have difficulty meeting your routine obligations? Is this real or only in your mind? Do your thoughts ever question your true purpose? Does the thought of doing what you really want seldom, if ever, occupy your thoughts? Is it safer to ignore the nagging idea to do something different for you and your family? If the answer is yes, you may be playing it safe.

Many of you already know that there is a greater purpose for your life and ignore the voices in your head. Purpose is your most valuable asset, and it will lead you where you really would like to be! Purpose can be the difference between success and failure. Purpose will keep you headed in the right direction, even if success may look like failure.

DON'T QUIT YOUR DAY JOB

So how can you test your purpose to decide if it's the real thing for you? This can be fairly easy and shouldn't complicate your life. Start by doing what you've dreamed about, to validate your perceived purpose. And here's an important point: Just because you believe you've found your purpose, don't quit your day job. At least not yet. You can test your purpose by taking side jobs (part-time) in your area of interest. Or you can volunteer your time to determine whether your purpose passes the test of time. If these efforts prove your thought process, it's time to make it real.

> Just because you believe you've found your purpose, don't quit your day job.

I have a friend who I've watched as she validates a new purpose in her life. She's been incredibly successful in the nonprofit world, working for several organizations in her professional career. She is very good at what she does and has derived a great deal of satisfaction throughout her career helping countless people along the way. Yet, there is something missing. She would like to transform the lives of people by introducing and instructing them in the world of plant-based nutrition, cooking, and eating. So in her free time, she's devoted countless hours to studying this field, taken various classes to advance her understanding of the topic, received numerous certifications in plant-based nutrition, and from a practical perspective, helped numerous individuals experience the benefits of this diet plan with fantastic results. She has dedicated the time to evaluate and determine if this is her real purpose, while maintaining her full-time position. The more she learns and understands this field, the more she realizes and confirms the true purpose of her life.

LIVE YOUR PURPOSE WITH PASSION

Purpose and passion are closely aligned. You can't have true purpose without the force of passion. Passion will ignite your life's purpose. You are the only one who can determine your purpose in your life because you define it. You are the only one who can combine your purpose with passion to find your version of success. When you understand your life's purpose, you will be exuberantly passionate about it. Finishing your race means understanding that it's never too late to find and live your purpose with passion. Ultimately, this will make a difference in yourself and others in your world. Find your purpose and live it with passion.

CHAPTER 10

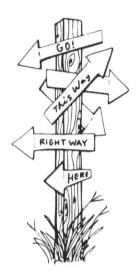

Discovering Your Direction: Setting Goals

"Setting goals is the first step in turning the invisible into the visible."

—Tony Robbins

Like most runners, I always have a finish time in mind when stepping up to the starting line of a race. On the morning of February 28, 2009, I was waiting for the start of the Cowtown Half Marathon with one goal in mind: to finish under two hours. It didn't matter if the finish line clock read 1:59:59, as long as I came in under two hours. Achieving this time goal would be a huge accomplishment, since two years earlier I'd completed my first post-cancer marathon in a time of 6:07:00 hours. That race, the 2007 Cowtown Marathon, represented a new challenge for me; I was eight months out from my last round of chemo and stem cell transplant, and I really wasn't sure how my body would hold up to 26.2 miles. On the day of this race, two years later, I felt fit and ready to go.

I had set my sub-two-hour time goal five months earlier. This seemed like a reasonable length of time to train my body and mind to achieve my target time. Every single training run was geared toward reaching this goal. My training plan included running several 5K (3.1 miles) races to gauge my progress and fitness. I passed these tests with flying colors. As a part of my race planning, I established specific time goals for every mile. I projected that if I could hit the intermediate times, I could hit my goal time. So, I set a specific goal with a time-line, wrote it down, developed a plan, and reviewed my progress on a regular basis. This is the same process you can use to realize any goal.

In the first few miles, I was able to hold my projected per-mile pace. By closely watching my mile split times along with projected 5K times, I was able to adjust my pace up or down to maintain a nine-minute-mile average pace. Everything was going as planned through about mile eight, when I heard a faint voice from behind me ask, "Can I run with you? I've been running behind you for about five miles, and I really like your pace." It's not unusual for a runner to focus on another runner's pace during a race. I had done it countless times, so of course I said, "Sure!"

I didn't know this person from the man in the moon, but over the next few miles we became friends. Funny how running together can have that result. She was from Dallas, had three daughters at home, and had left them with her husband so she could run her first half marathon. I was inspired by her story; she had been training on her own, sacrificing time with her family to accomplish something important to her, but this was also a teachable moment for her precious kids. She came to Fort Worth without any support, and she really wanted to achieve her goal to show her girls that you can do something if you set your mind to it. WOW! This sounded similar to my goal for this half marathon. At mile ten, I asked her if she had set a goal time. I will never forget her response. With a tear in her eye, she said, "I told my babies I would finish under two hours." What a coincidence! I glanced at my watch and quickly realized we could both achieve our goals, however, we had to step it up to make it happen. I told her, "Okay, we can do this, but we've got to pick up the pace."

As we got closer to the finish line, she fell behind me a couple of times. Each time she did, I encouraged her to maintain the pace. Several times, I literally felt like I was pulling her along with me. We were close to the two-hour mark and couldn't afford to slow down in these last miles. Finally, we turned the last corner, and the finish-line banner came into sight. I shouted to her, "Come on, you can do this!" As we crossed the finish line, I glanced at my watch and realized that we'd finished in under two hours. I turned back to my new friend to congratulate her as she collapsed into my arms in tears.

She was so relieved and excited, and so was I. We'd done it. I told her, "Tell your babies you finished in under two hours." She responded with a smile and a heartfelt "Thank you!"

GOAL SETTING WORKS!

As this story proves, setting goals works and can help you with so many aspects of your life by uniting purpose with action. You might be reading this and thinking, *"I've heard about the benefits of goal setting. But I've tried it. It just doesn't work!"* If that's you, I appreciate your response, and I understand your viewpoint. That's exactly why I wanted to include this chapter: to overcome that type of thinking. It's my belief that goal setting can be a huge plus in your life. It was an important part of my fight with cancer. After all, it was part of my old normal and would play an even bigger role in my "new" normal. I'd set goals my entire life with reliable, predictable results. Why couldn't it work with cancer?

> Setting goals works and can help you with so many aspects of your life by uniting purpose with action.

In the post-cancer treatment period, I decided to take a detailed, and what I considered unbiased, look at goal setting. What works, and what doesn't work? Why do different approaches seem successful while others always seem to fail? What constitutes a replicable, easy-to-follow goal-setting plan?

Here's what I discovered: First, goal setting might not have worked for you because it's never been fully explained to you. Second, many people think goal setting has to be complicated. It doesn't. Reliable goal setting is a simple, clearly defined process to help you achieve success. Third, there's a method and process to setting and achieving goals. Lastly, many people feel obligated rather than inspired by their goals, and that's often where the goal-setting disconnect occurs. Your goals have got to inspire you to take action. In other words, *Why* you set goals really counts.

So, has goal setting been something you've used in the past? Has it worked for you? If you want to consistently move forward in your life, goal setting will help you. It will empower you to take control of your life's direction, while providing you with benchmarks for determining whether you are actually succeeding.

Let's begin at *your* starting point and consider where *you* want to go. Yogi Berra, professional baseball catcher, manager, and coach said, "If you don't know where you are going, you'll end up somewhere else." So, where are you going? Instead of wandering through life on a day-to-day basis, figure out a game plan. Without goal setting, you will wind up, well, somewhere—it just might not be where you'd like to be. Setting a goal can help you find a destination and stay on track toward it. After all, how can you finish your race if you don't know where the course leads? Goals can serve as your road map. They provide clear, defined direction to your life. They offer you guidance and hold you accountable. Goals serve as well-defined targets coupled with a specific time frame and plan of action.

> Goals serve as well-defined targets coupled with a specific time frame and plan of action.

Along the journey, goals will help you determine what is and isn't important to you. The important things will stand out to you, while the less important things will fade with time. Distractions are often responsible for taking you off track in your life, but clearly defined goals can help to minimize distractions and open the way for a stronger decision-making process. Goals can take you places you've only dreamed of reaching.

GOAL SETTING MAKES A DIFFERENCE

Even though a lot of people are aware of the advantages of goal setting, few people consistently employ the process and even fewer do it with clarity of purpose. I'm not the only person who knows that it works. Studies have shown that 95% to 97% of the world's population does not set written goals. On the other hand, 3% to 5% of the world's population writes down their goals, and an even smaller percentage actually reaches them. A number of people in the 3% to 5% category don't succeed primarily due to a lack of seriousness and a general lack of understanding about what goal setting entails. These individuals may set goals, but they don't know how to achieve them via accomplishable steps. Some people set goals only once a year, like at New Year's, with little follow up. These goals seem like a good idea—it's something they do every year—but without a plan or a process to follow through, most of these goals are forgotten in short order. When the thrill of setting the goal is gone, so is the goal itself.

You are responsible for not only setting your goals but also for pursuing and achieving them to the fullest. And I won't mislead you: It takes work. In his 1984 book, *What They Don't Teach You at Harvard Business School*, Mark McCormack highlighted an often quoted and much debated 1979 Harvard study that observed the results of interviews with graduating MBA students.

- 3% of the MBA students had clear written goals and plans to accomplish them
- 13% had goals that were not committed to paper
- 84% had no specific goals at all

In 1989, ten years later, the same group of MBA students was interviewed again, with the following results:

- The 3% group, the one with written goals, earned ten times more than the other 97% put together.
- The 13% of the class who had goals (but not written) were earning, on average, twice as much as the 84% who had no goals at all.

Think this is by chance? I don't! Interestingly, even with ample evidence of goal-setting successes, the majority of individuals still don't have clear, specific, and written plans to work toward goals on an annual basis.

Dr. Edwin Locke is considered the pioneer of goal-setting theory. Starting in the 1960s, he devoted forty-plus years of his career to understanding the benefits and effects of goal setting on motivation. His extensive research efforts found that "for 90% of the time, specific and challenging (but not too challenging) goals lead to higher performance than easy, or 'do your best,' goals." In other words, you are more likely to be motivated and grow if you are challenged.

In a 1968 article, Locke proposed the theory that "working towards a goal provided a major source of motivation to actually reach the goal. The idea is that you become invested in reaching the goal, strengthening your motivation to achieve it." Locke found that individuals who set specific goals—difficult goals—performed better than those who set broad, easy goals. A more recent study conducted by Dr. Gail Matthews of Dominican University corroborated much of Dr. Locke's research, adding to the growing body of scientific data showing the correlation between effective goal setting and success. Her study primarily confirmed that individuals who write specific goals are more likely to consistently achieve them than those who have unwritten goals or no specific goals at all. Dr. Matthews added, "My study provides empirical evidence for the effectiveness of three coaching tools: accountability, commitment, and writing."

GOAL SETTING IS CRITICAL TO YOUR SUCCESS

Many people don't take goal setting seriously. Take New Year's resolutions, for instance. At this time of year, I know and under-stand that goals are set with the best intentions. I've made similar resolutions in the past with the same result: After a few weeks, I forgot about them. Goal setting should be taken seriously! Take Zig Ziglar's advice, if you don't believe me: "A goal casually set and lightly taken will be freely abandoned at the first obstacle." Often, New Year's resolutions come with no real, defined thinking process and no real emotion to motivate the goal setter to succeed. Effective goal setting can't be a one-time event. Instead, it's ongoing, forward-thinking, progressive, and never ends. It's a life-long process for your success.

Goal setting must be repetitious to be successful. Goal setting generally accompanies a change of some kind. A change is usually the result of developing a new habit. A habit results from the process of working toward a goal. Having a goal positively reinforces a new habit, giving you the ability to focus on accomplishing something specific. Focus results in efficiently and effectively using both your time and energy.

> Effective goal setting can't be a one-time event. Instead, it's ongoing, forward-thinking, progressive, and never ends. It's a life-long process for your success.

As a child, I was fascinated by the power of the sun and a magnifying glass. I would use a magnifying glass to aim a single beam of light on a piece of paper or wood. Once the beam was focused, smoke started to rise until the paper or wood was in flames due to the intensified power of the sun. This same type of result can be expected when you set a goal and concentrate your focus on achieving it.

Goals will get you out of your comfort zone—that's where your real progress happens. Goals should stretch and challenge you. As author and minister Gary Keesee says, "If you're not currently doing the hardest thing you've ever done, you're not growing."

Emotion is a goal-setting turbocharger. Goals must be set with emotion to promote meaning, substance, and desired results. You must have a strong *Why* (emotion) that energizes you to make a permanent change. Finally, accomplishing a goal almost always requires a positive, can-do attitude. A positive attitude keeps you motivated to pursue your goals with joy, excitement, and confidence.

GOAL SETTING IS A PROCESS

When it comes to setting goals, you first need to determine what you would like to achieve in life. What do you want to achieve today, in a month, in a year, in five years, in a lifetime? Goal setting quite often results from a desire to change some aspect of your life. How pressing is your desire to change? How compelled are you to change? Tony Robbins says, "Change happens when the pain of staying the same is greater than the pain of change." Does your need, want, or desire to change lead you to doing something monumental in your life?

Aim high. Challenge yourself. Think BIG! Own the goal! Reach for goals that excite and motivate you. That said, don't forget that your goals must be realistic and achievable. Ambitious goals are great, but they can't be *too* farfetched. Realistic goals are those within your skill set and level of accomplishment. Farfetched goals take you outside your knowledge base. You can't become an astronaut at the age of fifty, no matter how hard you try to convince yourself that you can. Unrealistic goals may be a source of frustration rather than motivation.

To achieve measurable success, you need a specific goal with a timeline and an action plan. During chemo, staying fit (as much as possible) while in the hospital was important to me. Yes, my body was subjected to incredibly harsh treatments. Yes, I was confined to the seventh floor of the hospital. Yes, I didn't have access to a gym. And yes, at times I didn't feel terrific. However, I could still do something for my physical fitness. This was within my power, and this was a goal I set!

So, on day one I made up my mind to walk every day to keep myself fit. Keep in mind, I didn't have access to a walking path or trail. The seventh floor is configured like a three-pointed star with three dead-end hallways. Okay, no problem. My goal was to walk one hour without stopping by the end of my stay. This meant walking everyday during, plus or minus the days when I physically couldn't. (This was my timeline.) I decided to walk once a day, mostly in the late afternoon, beginning with fifteen minutes (my action plan), increasing my time by two minutes (my intermediate goal) each day. My hospital stay was thirty-three days. I was walking an hour per day on my last day in the hospital. When I hit my goal, it wasn't long before I decided on a new one: running a marathon.

A WORD ABOUT FAILURE

Though this might surprise you, failure is an integral part of meeting a goal. Failure shows a concerted effort to meet a goal. You can and should learn from failure. Don't avoid setting goals just to avoid failure. Uncertainty often gets in the way of taking the first step toward achieving your goals. If fear holds you back, you're not alone. You might fear being judged by a failure, or you might fear that if you are unsuccessful at achieving a goal, others will be critical of you. As Thomas Edison said, "If I find 10,000 ways something won't work, I haven't failed. I'm not discouraged because every wrong attempt discarded is often a step forward."

The best tool against fear is action. Once you've set your goals, just go ahead and dive in. Take that first step. Chances are you'll feel far better than you did before you got started. Be confident that one step leads to another. Look for reasons you'll succeed (and you will!), not reasons you can't succeed. And if, after everything, you've set goals that seem

> Look for reasons you'll succeed (and you will!), not reasons you can't succeed.

unrealistic, you can revise them. Don't give up on your dream just because you're not yet headed in the direction you want. There can be different routes to the same destination.

GOAL-SETTING STEP 1: SET SPECIFIC GOALS

It's time to set some goals of your own. First off, when it comes to goal setting, it is important to be specific. By specific, I mean quantitative. Goals that are vague are often difficult to achieve and give you plenty of reasons to get off track. Describe your goal in detail, the more specific the better. If you decide to make losing weight a goal, it's not enough to say, "I am going to lose weight this year." This won't work because it leaves too much out of the equation. Instead, you've got to quantify this goal by saying, "I will lose fifty pounds by June 30. I will eliminate sugar from my diet and eat three balanced meals each day. In addition, I will exercise three days per week for one hour each session." Dr. Edwin Locke's research showed that the more difficult and specific a goal is, the harder you tend to work to achieve it.

To maintain your goal, it must spark or pique your interest. If you feel a spark, it will make an impact on your ability to stick with it and work toward your goal. A spark can lead to excitement, and excitement can motivate you. If you're motivated, your goal may change your life. That's what achieving goals is all about! And if you don't feel strongly about a particular goal, you might need to reconsider it, replacing it with one that holds your interest and motivates you.

It is absolutely vital to consider *Why* your goal is important to you. *Why* is it of value to you? *Why* will accomplishing it will improve your life? This simple step is often forgotten and often results in disappointment. So, provide sufficient reasons to make the goal real and achievable. Clearly define *Why* you want to achieve this goal. For a weight-loss goal, your reasons might include

> Clearly define Why you want to achieve this goal.

improved health, greater self-esteem, and more physical endurance. Holding your *Why* in your mind and coming back to it when you reach an obstacle may very well make the difference between success and failure. The stronger your *Why*, the stronger your commitment to success.

Finally, it is important to consider the consequences of not achieving a goal. Not achieving your weight-loss goal could potentially lead to a serious illness in the future, the need to take medications (blood pressure, cholesterol meds, etc.), an inability to be as active as you'd like, and more. So, take the time to consider the "what if" scenarios, if you don't achieve a goal. Recognizing the potential results of failing to reach a goal can have a significant impact on actually achieving a goal and can lead to the greatest moments of success!

GOAL-SETTING STEP 2: SELECT A DEADLINE FOR GOAL COMPLETION

It's important to set a defined deadline, including a start date and a completion date. Choose a specific day, month, and year. Next week or by the end of the year isn't good enough. Without a deadline, there is no motivation to achieve a goal. A deadline creates a sense of urgency, gives you a chance to evaluate your progress as time passes, and is measurable. As Peter Drucker, author, educator, and management consultant said, "If you can't measure it, you can't improve it." So, be committed with a sense of urgency and decide, "I will achieve this goal!"

GOAL-SETTING STEP 3: WRITE DOWN YOUR GOAL

Goals that are written, particularly in your handwriting, make you more accountable to the goal. If your goals are not written, they are destined to be only dreams. Writing out a goal makes it real and tangible! Committing goals to paper and reviewing them regularly gives you a 95% higher chance of achieving your desired outcomes. Studies have verified that writing down your goals puts you in the top 3% of the world population of goal achievers. Remember Dr. Gail Matthews' study: "Those who wrote their goals accomplished significantly more than those who did not write their goals."

> Goals that are written, particularly in your handwriting, make you more accountable to the goal.

Writing your goals helps you to visualize the end result and serves to focus or motivate your efforts. It's not enough to think about achieving something. You've got to turn your thoughts into real, tangible targets, giving them meaning and providing momentum for success.

GOAL-SETTING STEP 4: DEVELOP A PLAN AND COMMIT TO IT

Develop a detailed plan with clear steps to achieve your goals. This will serve as your road map. Plan your way to success! Your plan must be realistic, and you should be willing to commit to it with an overwhelming desire to achieve the goal. In other words, you must be willing to dedicate the time and effort required to complete each step of your plan, which might mean making adjustments in other aspects of your life. As Thomas Jefferson, third president of the United States, said, "If you want something you've never had, you must be willing to do something you've never done before."

Your plan should include short-, medium-, and long-term goals. Short-term goals are the critical steps you take to accomplish your medium-term goals. Achieving a medium-term goal leads to completing a long-term goal. Remember, a marathon is 26.2 miles, but you run it one step at a time, one mile at a time, until you cross the finish line. But each step counts. You must take a series of small steps to achieve your giant leap.

Almost every goal will benefit from setting milestones along the way to your completion date. Depending on the timeline of your goal, you should set short-, medium-, and long-term milestones. Set milestones at a minimum of one week, one month, six months, and one year. Set extended milestones at five years, ten years, and a lifetime. By setting and achieving these milestones, you will gain a sense of accomplishment and confidence as you strive to reach your ultimate goal. When training for a marathon, I set intermediate training goals. Twelve weeks out, I run fourteen miles; nine weeks from the event, I run sixteen miles; six weeks from the event, I run eighteen miles; and three weeks from the event, I run twenty miles, which takes me right up to event day ready for the marathon. If I hit those milestones, I have confidence that I will be prepared to cross the finish line.

GOAL-SETTING STEP 5: REVIEW YOUR GOAL(S) EVERY DAY

Setting specific, written goals combined with a clearly defined plan to achieve success is paramount; however, you absolutely must review your goals on a regular basis. Reviewing your goals provides a useful reality check for you. Over the long term, your situation may change, so allow yourself the flexibility to revise or modify your goals and the action plan. Keep in mind that your goals were based on your situation when you first set them.

Read or write your goals twice a day, in the morning to motivate you and in the evening to renew your mind. Motivation to reach your goal is enough to get you started, however, as discussed, repetition leads to a habit, and habit will keep you going. It generally takes twenty-one to thirty days to form a habit. Within a month, reviewing your goals should become automatic. As previously mentioned, less than 3% of Americans have written goals, and of those who do, less than 1% review and revise their goals on a regular basis. This means as soon as you start setting goals and reviewing them regularly, you'll be ahead of 99% of the general population.

The process of measuring your daily progress should provide clarity, focus, and a sense of accomplishment when you reach your short- and medium-term goals. Lao Tzu, considered to be the founder of Taoism, is quoted as saying, "People usually fail when they are on the verge of success. So give as much care to the end as to the beginning: Then there will be no failure." Remember, reviewing your goals daily will keep you on the path to achieving them!

> Remember, reviewing your goals daily will keep you on the path to achieving them!

READY, SET, GOAL

There will never be a "right time" to start setting goals! You can make excuses about how and when you're going to start, to feel better about letting yourself off the hook, but you're only kidding yourself if you take that approach. Start now, follow the steps outlined in this chapter, and turn your dreams into reality.

CHAPTER 11

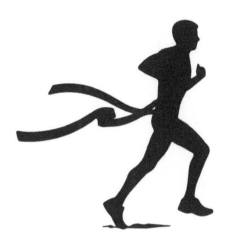

The Power of Action

"The distance between dreams and reality is called action."

—Unknown

It is not enough to have a dream or set a goal. Formulating a plan to achieve your dream or goal doesn't magically make it happen. Every accomplishment in the world started as an idea. Someone had to be willing to do something to turn the idea into reality. That something is action! Without action, dreams or goals remain just that—dreams or goals.

> Without action, dreams or goals remain just that—dreams or goals.

At 211 degrees, water is hot. At 212 degrees, it boils. One extra degree makes all the difference. That extra degree does not come automatically. It has to be applied by turning on the heat. That extra degree corresponds to your action. The one extra degree of action in every aspect of your life can turn a dream, goal, or idea into reality. It only takes one degree to make a difference. As straightforward and easy as an additional one degree may sound, you have to make this happen. Action is up to you!

Prior to cancer, I was always waiting for the right time, the right moment, some sign, signal, or catalyst before I would get started. I would wish, hope, and pray for something to happen. My race with cancer showed me that the right time is *now*. The right time is always right in front of you. The power was (and still is) within me, as it is within you. You simply have to turn on your heat and take action.

Joyce Meyer, a Christian author and speaker, put the concept of action this way: "If you don't want to have regrets later, then now is the time to take action, not tomorrow, not next year, not when you feel like it, not when it's convenient—now is the time to take action."

WHAT'S IN A WORD?

Action is defined as "the process or state of acting or of being active; something done or performed; act; deed." Applying action leads to results. Action brings a goal to fruition, leads to solutions for a problem, and turns adversity around, resulting in more predictable successes. With action, everything you think, believe, and hope for can and will be accomplished. You must be willing to take action to move forward. Once again, it's up to you!

> Action brings a goal to fruition, leads to solutions for a problem, and turns adversity around, resulting in more predictable successes.

Thomas Edison, who is credited with inventing the electric lightbulb, is a great example of the power of action. He was not the only person working on inventing the first affordable incandescent lightbulb for use in the home. However, he was the first to refine the lightbulb and make it available to the masses. This did not come without a lot of action. Edison was looking for the best filament for the lightbulb, something that was durable and inexpensive. He and his team tested more than six thousand materials before finding one that consistently worked—carbonized bamboo. Discovering the proper filament was essential to Edison's success. The relentless effort he and his team made to find it is what counts. He could have easily stopped the search and declared enough was enough at any moment along the way. However, he didn't! Action, his relentless effort, was the watchword that kept him going. Edison had an idea, applied action, and the rest is history!

THE IMPORTANCE OF ACTION

Is action the watchword that keeps you going when times are tough or you're looking for inspiration and motivation? Any successful journey you take in your life will start with action and end with action.

Choosing to take action is the first step in any journey. You've got to start somewhere! You must move past thinking and start doing. This is the power of action. Taking action sounds easy enough, but it's easier said than done. You've got to have courage to take action, and believe me there are plenty of distractions that will stand in your way.

Once you take action to reach a goal, solve a problem, or turn adversity into a positive, you can't stop the momentum. Like Edison, your actions must be consistent and persistent to achieve success. To make this happen, determine the single action you need to take every day to bring you one step closer to success. Apply this action every day, every week, every month without exception to achieve your objective. Be mindful that to be successful, you've got to apply action no matter how you feel physically, mentally, or emotionally: good, bad, or indifferent. There will certainly be times when you won't want to take action, and these are the times that you must. You can achieve success in spite of your how badly you feel or the circumstances surrounding your life—if you take action!

Here's something I've discovered that has been invaluable to me: Success in life generally requires some sort of change. If you want to lose weight, you've got to change the way you eat. If you want to become physically fit, you've got to start working out. If you want to be the best in your professional field, you've got to work hard to understand every aspect of the job. If you want to create better relationships with others, you've got to make this a priority and commit to making it happen. You can't expect the desired outcome to simply fall into your lap without any effort. As author Catherine Pulsifer says, "No action, no change. Limited action, limited change. Lots of action, change occurs." Nothing will change without action. Tony Robbins reminds us, "If you do what you've always done, you'll get what you've always gotten."

Success and change go hand in hand. You've almost always got to change something in your life to experience success. Sometimes it's only one thing, one thought, or one extra effort that makes the difference and gets you over the top. Action is the catalyst for the change that leads to success. You've got an inherent need to succeed. I believe it's a part of our nature and in our DNA to be successful. However, not all of us reach the same level of success. Why is that? We are simply not all built the same way, and we certainly don't all have the same life experiences when it comes to the concept of success. As a result, we don't all look at the road to success from the same viewpoint. We also don't all have the tools to overcome the obstacles that invariably get in the way of success.

> The formula is simple: Action equals change equals success.

Honestly, many people are not always *willing* to take action to change—me included. The formula is simple: Action equals change equals success.

DISTRACTIONS CAN STOP YOUR ACTION

I don't profess to be a psychologist, but my battle with cancer has taught me that we often surrender to distractions. I had plenty of distractions during my journey that could have easily derailed my road to recovery. Side effects were a common part of chemo from day one, and believe me I had my share. It wasn't unusual for me to have an upset stomach, feel tired, and at times have no desire to do anything. These distractions could have slowed my recovery, except I didn't let that happen. I chose to get busy physically and mentally, in spite of how I felt. This wasn't always possible, but it was certainly my daily mantra.

I experience distractions, like most of you, at some level every day, and I know from plenty of personal and professional experience that distractions can keep you from achieving your highest level of success. That's why it pays to be aware of the distractions that most often affect you—in order to overcome them. Distractions take on many forms, but, from my perspective, let me break down the two main types: simple (external) and complex (internal).

Simple distractions are those that generally require—or seem like they require—our immediate attention. A coworker walks into your office, the phone rings as you're putting the finishing touches on a project, your boss calls an unplanned meeting, there's a knock at your door, the familiar ding of an incoming email, and so on. These distractions can occur at work or home and the list goes on: email, Twitter, Facebook, a baby crying to be fed, a dog whining to be let out, a neighbor coming over unexpectedly, express mail arrival at your door, etc. Enough already! Simple distractions are often unexpected and unpredictable. Fortunately, they are generally brief. However, many (or most) of these are time wasters, which can disrupt concentration and result in a loss of momentum. It takes only a moment to be distracted, but it can take much longer to get back on track.

Complex distractions, on the other hand, are generally self-induced and originate in our minds. These distractions have a tendency to result in self-sabotage and often keep us from succeeding. There is a long list of these distractions: fear, including fear of failure, fear of success, fear of the unknown, fear of change, and fear of rejection. Additional complex distractions include doubt, worry, uncertainty, insecurity, memories, experiences, and procrastination.

> It takes only a moment to be distracted, but it can take much longer to get back on track.

Complex distractions can become excuses and can ultimately take control over our ability or inability to be successful. In other words, complex distractions can limit our beliefs, sabotaging progress and, ultimately, our future. If you've used one or more of the excuses below, consciously or unconsciously, distractions have impacted your ability to succeed. Welcome to the crowd, I am right there with you!

- I can't do that.
- I'm not smart enough.
- I don't have the proper education.
- I don't know the right person.
- I am not qualified.
- I am overqualified.
- I'm too young.

- ◆ I'm too old.
- ◆ I don't have the time.
- ◆ I don't have enough money.

The impact of distractions can be short term, as is the case with most simple distractions, or long term, especially for those more complex distractions. Bottom line, distractions stop your progress and keep you from becoming all you are capable of being.

FEAR OF FAILURE—DISTRACTION

A few more important words about one of the most prevalent distractions—fear of failure. The word "failure" often has negative connotations in our society. It's important to recognize that failure is an unavoidable part of life. More than likely, if you're not failing, you're not testing yourself enough. In fact, it's unrealistic to expect that you won't fail. If you don't fail, you will never learn. If you never learn, you will never change. If you don't learn from your failures, you're destined to repeat them again and again.

I experienced the concept of failure at a young age as I learned the game of golf. Failing was my best teacher. I chose to look at my failures as opportunities to learn. As a result, my golf game improved every time that I understood why I failed. Don't get me wrong—no one wants to fail. Certainly, no one strives to fail. I'm sure that none of you wake up in the morning hoping to fail. Still, it is important to understand that there are valuable lessons in failing, which are essential to learning. Failure gives you a second (and a third, fourth, fifth, etc.) chance to learn from your mistakes and do the right thing the next time. Here's an important point to consider, failure is not final unless you refuse to try again. There is almost always a next time so take advantage of the opportunity to try again.

Failure tests our resolve and builds character. If viewed in a positive manner, failing forces us to adapt and change. Failure can be your route to success because failure and success are

> Failure is not final unless you refuse to try again.

so closely related. You tip the scales in favor of success when you make the decision to succeed. It's your choice to turn failure into success. As entrepreneur and author Gary Keller says, "Extraordinary results are rarely happenstance! They come from the choices we make and the actions we take!" Failure can lead you to the greatest successes of your life provided you approach it with a positive attitude.

Let me be clear, failure is not a substitute for success. It's something you should try to avoid. More often than not, failure is a short-lived obstacle on the more meaningful journey of your life. Everyone, without exception, will experience failure at one point or another. Many of you will come across failure numerous times. I know that I have! What truly matters is how you react to and learn from that failure. Failure should motivate you to new heights.

There are countless examples of success stories in American history that started as failures. These people are perfect examples of why failure should never, ever stop you from following your dream. Walt Disney, pioneer of the American animation industry, was fired from the newspaper he worked for in 1919 because, he was told, he "lacked imagination and had no good ideas." This failure was followed by others, including several business ventures which ended in misfortunes. Disney did not give up and went on to create one of the most successful cartoon characters ever in Mickey Mouse. He went on to be one of the most creative geniuses of the twentieth century. He could have succumbed to failure and given up. Instead, he chose to use failure as a catalyst to succeed.

I'm reminded of a quote by Rick Warren, evangelical Christian pastor and author: "Failure is never final. You're never a failure until you quit, and it's always too soon to quit. You don't determine a person's greatness by his talent, his wealth, or his education. You determine a person's greatness by what it takes to discourage him." There may not be a better description of the word "failure."

EVALUATING DISTRACTIONS IN YOUR LIFE

If you are like me, from time to time distractions have gotten you off track and made a significant impact on your life. It is difficult, if not impossible, to avoid this possibility. Distractions can keep you from achieving a goal, solving a problem, or overcoming adversity. Heck, distractions can keep you from getting out the door in the morning in order to make it to work on time.

Let's consider distractions in your life. You might want to have a pen and paper ready to jot your thoughts down. It's essential to consider and identify the distractions that hold you back from success. What can you define as distractions that keep you from realizing a goal? Which distractions have the most significant impact on your life? For me, that's relatively easy: A simple distraction would be email and social media; a complex distraction would be fear of failure.

Listen, listing my known distractions was not easy to do. Yes, admitting to these distractions is difficult. I struggle with these distractions (and others) every single day. However, recognition of my distractions helps me overcome them and move forward. For me, distractions get me off track and lead to procrastination. In spite of the procrastination, I know where I'm headed and why, and eventually I will get there. However, distractions make this process far harder than it needs to be. In the process of writing this book, for example, very often I would get on a roll while writing a chapter, but from time to time my uncertainty about a specific message would lead me to check my emails, look at Facebook, or make an unrelated phone call in the name of "I've got to do these things!" Quite often, these distractions would get me off track and delay the inevitable, which was completing the section on which I was working.

For me, distractions often become excuses or justifications that slow my progress toward achieving a goal. I will, at times, use these excuses to justify my lack of progress. For some reason, there is a bit of comfort in this type of justification, allowing me to stay in my comfort zone.

Have you ever gotten on a roll with a work or home project only to yield to distractions? You are excited and headed for success and, invariably, you get in your own way. Are you your own worst enemy when it comes to distractions that sabotage your success? This is the time to come face to face with your distractions. Don't ignore them!

Be honest with yourself. Take positive action and overcome the distractions. Evaluating and understanding your specific distractions will make you better equipped to achieve success in all areas of your life. Trust this process—it will make a difference!

FOCUS: OVERCOMING YOUR DISTRACTIONS—STAYING ON TRACK!

So far in this chapter, you've been introduced to the power and benefits of action. You've read how distractions hold you back from taking action. You've even identified some of your distractions. But even with this new knowledge base, what if distractions still get the best of you? How can you make the power of action an unstoppable reality and get things done in your life? In one word: "Focus!"

If there's power in action, there's clarity, direction, and success in focus. Focus means concentrating solely on one specific item or task at a time. Society today seems to reward or even revere individuals who can multitask. In fact, many of you take great pride in believing you are a natural at multitasking, as if this is some kind of skill. However, here's the truth: It's been shown that the human mind can actually only do one thing well at a time. Yet, if you are an accomplished multitasker, you find yourself trying to do more than one thing at a time.

> If there's power in action, there's clarity, direction, and success in focus.

In an effort to multitask, your brain switches from one task to another. In this effort, the brain is forced to reset to the new task.

Generally, this process results in none of the tasks being completed in a timely or successful manner. In addition, because you don't listen as well when multitasking, quite often mistakes are made, misunderstandings are created, and results may be less than satisfactory. Focusing on one task for a sufficient time can make a significant impact on the quality of your work, including how quickly it's completed and what thoughts or ideas are generated from completing each task mindfully. As life coach Mark Ferguson says, "When you focus on one task or one thought, you create a much better result in every aspect of your life."

DISTRACTION-PROOF YOUR LIFE

Let's face it, none of us are free from distractions. This is a fact of life. Simple distractions are easier to deal with than complex distractions. Simple distractions are dealt with by pushing past the interruption. Complex distractions are a bit more complicated and require a more focused effort. Focus is essential to your long-term success. Tony Robbins says, "You get what you focus on." Understand that focus is hard and takes work.

Here are a few steps you can take to achieve focus in your day-to-day activities:

- ◆ Plan your day ahead of time. This concept is paramount. Select either the night or the morning for your planning period. Your plan will define the tasks for the day ahead and will serve as a checklist of the tasks to be completed. I like to make my plan the night before so I can hit the ground running when I start my day. Focus on what you need to accomplish during the day to consider it a success. Keep your plan in front of you throughout the day.

- Find a comfortable, quiet place to work. Whether in your office away from home or your home office, you need a good desk and chair along with the appropriate equipment to complete your tasks.

- Define a specific work time frame. For me, that's one hour. In that time frame, I will focus on the task at hand. At the end of that time frame, I take a five or ten minute break before I get started again. By working nonstop, uninterrupted for one hour, I don't feel guilty about taking a short break.

- Control your office environment as much as possible. In other words, close the door or the shutters while working. This will eliminate visual distractions.

- Avoid answering the phone within your established work time frame. For me, I've got to turn off the phone and any other device which can serve as a distraction.

- Do not check email within your established work time frame.

- Ignore social media of any kind within your established work time frame, including Facebook, Twitter, Instagram, etc.

THE FREEDOM OF FOCUS

Make focusing a consistent and persistent activity, and try to avoid multitasking if possible. Complete one task at a time within a specific time frame before moving on to the next thing. Focusing can and should be a conscious activity that factors into your day-to-day planning process. It's okay to say, *"I've got to focus on this task today, even if that means I won't get to this other task."* As you get better at the act of focusing, this should become a habit you use every single day.

I've had numerous occasions to use focus in my life, both before and after cancer. In the early 2000s, I made the decision to change careers and entered the financial services industry. This required me to acquire several qualifying licenses. I'd been fairly good at taking tests in the past, but, this was a different challenge—financial services were a totally new ball game for me, with all new skills to learn. Obtaining the Series 7 license was imperative, as it allows the holder to sell all types of securities products. In addition, the firm I chose to work with made it clear that passing the Series 7 exam was not an option—it was a must to remain employed. However, in the process of interviewing me and encouraging me to become a part of the team, they didn't exactly communicate the urgency of taking and passing this demanding test. No big deal, right? Wrong! I soon learned that I had to pass the exam within three months, or I would be immediately terminated.

I knew what I had to do. My attention was on taking action and focusing on the task at hand. The stakes were high! Nothing could get in the way of my acquiring this license. I came up with an overall study plan and picked a time frame to complete my studies. At the end of every day, I developed a study plan for the next day. I studied in my home office knowing I could close the door and shutters, keeping out any unwanted guests. I set up study hours and limited all interruptions that might keep me from studying. I made passing the Series 7 a priority (like a job) and didn't let anything keep me from being prepared. I studied three months for this exam, a minimum of eight hours a day. At the end of this time frame, I was ready. I passed the exam on my first attempt. Action followed by focus got the job done.

> If you want to make things happen in your life on a more consistent basis, make focus an integral part of everything you do.

If you want to make things happen in your life on a more consistent basis, make focus an integral part of everything you do. Focus will help you overcome distractions, keep you on track, help you complete tasks faster with higher quality, and lead to greater success in all areas of your life. There is freedom in focus!

ACTION WITH FOCUS IN YOUR LIFE

If you've been frustrated or discouraged by how hard it can seem to overcome distractions, you are not alone. I am certain many of you, like me, share in this frustration. It's important to focus on what you are striving to achieve, NOT the distractions (excuses) that keep you from being successful. So many of us place too much attention and emphasis on the distractions and not on the best ways to focus and overcome distractions. Are you focused on your goal and the steps that lead you to success? Or are you allowing distractions to receive far too much of your attention?

Action can do a lot to make positive outcomes possible in your life. Action gets you started. Focus keeps you moving in a positive direction toward achievement. Focusing on a consistent basis is easier said than done because of the distractions we encounter every day. You must diligently work against distractions and towards focus to achieve positive results.

A few final reminders and tips about focus:

- In an effort to free yourself from distractions, create an environment that allows you to focus. Where (or what) is your most productive environment?
- Take on one task or project at a time. Prioritize your tasks.
- Set aside a specific amount of time to focus on a task, and make your best effort to avoid distractions.
- Focus on what you are striving to achieve, NOT the distractions (excuses) that keep you from being successful.
- When you feel frustrated or discouraged about your lack of progress toward a goal, remember your *Why* to move forward again.

Applying action is an important ingredient in making things happen in your life. Whether you are trying to achieve a goal or are faced with a problem, the most significant thing you can do is get busy by taking action. So many people identify a goal, problem, or challenge, and then sit and wait for things to get better or change on their own. That was my method of operation for years! The world doesn't work that way. Only by making things happen can you realize change. Action is the way to change your situation and impact your outcome for the better!

CONCLUSION

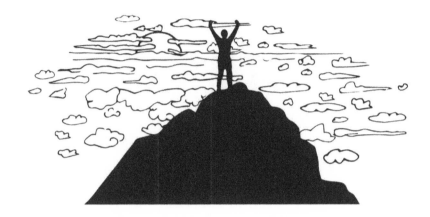

Finish Your Race

"Each day is a new beginning."

—Michael Duff Newton

A couple of days before my first one hundred-mile cycle event at "America's Most Beautiful Bike Ride" in Lake Tahoe in early June 2016, a friend asked me how I was feeling about my upcoming century ride. I shared with him that I wished I had completed a few more training rides in preparation for the event. In response, he said, "I get it! I know you're extremely competitive and always want to do your very best." Shaking his head up and down, he reminded me of something that really got my attention. He said, "Remember how far you've come and all you've done in the last ten years." His comment certainly put things in perspective for me and made me stop and think. Thoughts of the previous ten years flashed in my mind. Some bad, but mostly good! He was so right; I had come a long way in what seemed like a short amount of time. I am a survivor transforming to a "thriver" in life.

Eleven years ago, I was diagnosed with a disease that could have taken my life. This was a pivotal moment in my life—what an understatement! I could have succumbed to the disease or, as I did, fight with every fiber of my body to live. For me, every day since my recovery has been a new beginning and an opportunity to discover my true, authentic, improved self.

This journey, my race of self-discovery, was not always comfortable for me. I found that my life was out of whack in so many ways: priorities, motivations, goals, and more. I was successful in business but not necessarily in other areas of my life. I had missed out on so much that life had to offer. I concentrated far too much on me instead of my relationships with others and the world around me. It's difficult for me to even think or verbalize that thought, but it's good that I've come far enough to recognize it. This understanding has led me to who I am today and thrust me in a new direction for my life. It may be difficult for others to comprehend but, for me on a very personal level, leukemia was the best thing that ever happened to me. It changed my priorities and opened my eyes to a purpose far bigger than myself or anything I could have imagined.

My cancer journey was filled with uncertainty and doubt about my future. My victory over cancer led me to a renewed understanding about life, resulting in new lessons and, ultimately, strategies that allowed me to change every aspect of my life. However, these strategies are not unique to just me; everyone can use them to empower their lives.

Since my recovery from cancer, I've been on a mission to make a difference in my life and, more importantly, the lives of others by sharing my experiences. I hope this book has been helpful and useful in the way you manage and conduct the various areas of your life. My endeavor in writing this book has been to equip you with life strategies to find, or rekindle, your purpose, which, when combined with an unstoppable passion, can help you be more successful on your own terms.

It is my desire that this book has been an inspiration for you and, in some small way, motivates you to make changes in your life and find your race, a race that will lead to incredible, meaningful outcomes now and in the future. It's important for you to realize that just reading this book alone will not have a meaningful impact on your life. You've got to take action based on your self-discoveries. The good news is, you don't have to wait for that perfect moment to start taking action. You can start taking action toward your best life right now.

My journey with leukemia revealed to me so many important

facets of life which I never considered. I've embraced these themes in this book. Here's a recap of the themes I covered:

- **Adversity** affects all of us at one time or another. It's not the adversity itself, but how we react to it that can define and change the direction and outcome of our lives.

- **Attitude** is a game changer. By changing your attitude, you can change your life and determine the course of your future.

- **Balance** is an important concept to be aware of, as it affects so many areas of our lives: work, play, relationships, and more. However, don't obsess about life balance. Instead be conscious of how life balance affects yourself and others. Learn to be flexible in applying this concept to your daily life.

- **Expectations** are derived from your life experiences from the day you were born and affect every area of your life. Expectations are powerful enough to influence your perception of an outcome, both good and not so good.

- **Purpose** is a powerful motivator in your life, providing meaning and direction to every waking hour of the day. Purpose and passion are not the same, yet they are inseparable. Purpose is your reason and passion is the energy which powers the way.

- **Goal setting** can make a difference in your life. I'm not talking about New Year's resolutions. I am talking about a process that works and leads to your success.

- **Action** is the catalyst that can make an idea a reality, the relentless effort that can solve a problem, and the ingredient that can bring a goal to fruition. Distractions, of all types, can and do slow or stop your actions. Focus combined with action can help you overcome distractions and lead to even quicker and more meaningful success.

Setbacks can affect all of our lives. The setback for me, which led to the writing of this book, was leukemia. Setbacks in your life may appear in the form of illness, job loss, bankruptcy, divorce, the death of a loved one, and more. Maybe you're experiencing one of those setbacks right now, and you don't know how and why it began or what to do next. It is my hope, as you finish this book that you will be equipped with strategies to empower your life and overcome any setback you encounter.

We are all survivors of something, and though it may not feel like it now, you will get through any setback that comes your way—I DID and so can YOU! Although there are no guarantees in life, and everything you know can change in the blink of an eye, remember that you are always responsible for yourself and the outcome of your life. So take the first step to move forward in your life.

Don't do what I did and wait for a life-threatening event to make you stop and take inventory of your life and its direction. Each and every day, you have the choice to influence your future and, in the process, impact the outcome of your life and the lives of those around you. You have the power to make choices which yield meaningful, positive victories in your life and others. And you can start NOW! Life is full of victories, you just have to claim them – one by one!

Every day presents an opportunity to choose to be positive and successful in your own way. I wouldn't want anyone to go through what I did with cancer. However, if there's one thing you can learn from my experience, it's this:

It's *never* too late to make a difference in yourself and others. With courage, focus, and a positive spirit, you *can* discover, or rediscover, what living your best life means to you.

So what are you waiting for? Get out there, get started and ***Finish YOUR Race!***

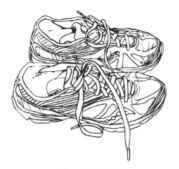

RACE
RESOURCES

Several organizations were important to me during my race with leukemia. Each of these organizations played a specific and vital role in my survival. Collectively, they were the team that got me across the finish line. I am forever grateful for this team and their extraordinary efforts.

I would like you to know more about these invaluable nonprofits and hospitals and the roles they may play in a cancer patient's journey. Please take the time to check out these resources on the pages ahead. If you ever need support, you've got a place to call.

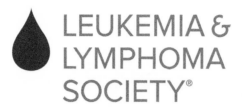

LEUKEMIA & LYMPHOMA SOCIETY®

fighting blood cancers

The **Leukemia & Lymphoma Society (LLS)** is the world's largest voluntary health agency dedicated to blood cancer. The LLS mission: Cure leukemia, lymphoma, Hodgkin's disease and myeloma, and improve the quality of life of patients and their families. LLS funds lifesaving blood cancer research around the world and provides free information and support services. LLS exists to find cures and ensure access to treatments for blood cancer patients. We are the voice for all blood cancer patients and we work to ensure access to treatments for all blood cancer patients.

www.lls.org

BE ✿ THE MATCH®

For people with life-threatening blood cancers—like leukemia and lymphoma—or other diseases, a cure exists. **Be The Match** connects patients with their donor match for a life-saving marrow or umbilical cord blood transplant. Be The Match provides patients and their families one-on-one support, education, and guidance before, during and after transplant You can help save a life as a committed member of the Be The Match Registry® , financial contributor or volunteer. To learn more about the cure, visit BeTheMatch.org or call 1 (800) MARROW-2.

BeTheMatch.org

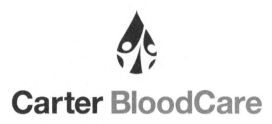

Carter BloodCare

Carter BloodCare's primary purpose is to make blood transfusions available for hospital patients within its regional service area. The blood center is a not-for-profit, 501(c) 3 organization that recruits blood donors, collects blood from volunteer donors; processes, tests and distributes the blood products to more than 200 medical facilities in more than 55 counties. Headquarters and service areas are located in north, central and east Texas. To make an appointment, call 1-800-DONATE-4 (800-366-2834) or visit www.carterbloodcare.org. The blood program is licensed by the U.S. Food and Drug Administration, accredited by AABB and is a member of America's Blood Centers.

www.carterbloodcare.org

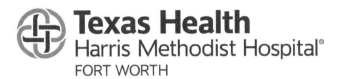

The Klabzuba Cancer Center at Texas Health Harris Methodist Hospital Fort Worth provides quality care throughout the cancer journey. The program's vision of striving for a future without cancer is reflected in its continuum of services: prevention, screening, early detection, treatment planning, surgery, chemotherapy, radiation, rehabilitation, palliative care and more.

The cancer center received the "Outstanding Achievement Award" from the Commission on Cancer (CoC) of the American College of Surgeons for excellence in the key areas of patient care. This demonstrates the high quality care provided to Texas Health Fort Worth patients from diagnosis, through the treatment period, and beyond.

TexasHealth.org/FW-Cancer

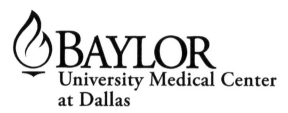

BAYLOR
University Medical Center at Dallas

Baylor Charles A. Sammons Cancer Center

Part of ✚BaylorScott&White HEALTH

For nearly four decades, **Baylor Charles A. Sammons Cancer Center**, an integral part of Baylor University Medical Center at Dallas, has provided quality clinical care, advanced technology, and clinical research to patients, along with comprehensive support services and programs for patients and their families. With the opening of a 10-story outpatient treatment facility and integration with Baylor T. Boone Pickens Cancer Hospital, it is now the largest outpatient cancer center in North Texas. Annually, more than 90,000 cancer visits occur at Baylor Sammons Cancer Center, and more than 800 people participate in research trials.

BaylorScottandWhite.com

CPSIA information can be obtained
at www.ICGtesting.com
Printed in the USA
LVHW110125110219
606938LV00001BB/2/P